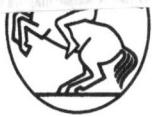

N. Kolev, G. Huemer, M. Zimpfer

Transesophageal Echocardiography

A New Monitoring Technique

Springer-Verlag Wien GmbH

Nikolai Kolev, MD, FACC
Research Cardiologist Associate in Anesthesia and
Consultant Echocardiographer, Firma Hewlett Packard
Department of Anesthesiology and General Intensive Care,
University of Vienna, Austria

Günter Huemer, MD
Staff Anesthesiologist
Department of Anesthesiology and General Intensive Care,
University of Vienna, Austria

Michael Zimpfer, MD
Professor of Anesthesia
Chairman of the Department of Anesthesiology and
General Intensive Care, University of Vienna, Austria

© 1995 Springer-Verlag Wien
Originally published by Springer-Verlag/Wien in 1995

Typesetting and Data-conversion: Thomson Press, India

Printed on acid-free and chlorine-free bleached paper

With 77 partly coloured Figures

Library of Congress Cataloging-in-Publication Data.

Kolev, N. (Nikolai), 1942– . Transesophageal echocardiography: a new monitoring technique / N. Kolev, G. Huemer, M. Zimpfer. p. cm.
ISBN 978-3-211-82650-8   ISBN 978-3-7091-7676-4 (eBook)
DOI 10.1007/978-3-7091-7676-4

1. Transesophageal echocardiography. I. Huemer G. (Günter). II. Zimpfer, M. (Michael), 1951– . III. Title.
[DNLM: 1. Echocardiography, Transesophageal. WG 141.5.E2 K81t 1994].
RC683.5.T83K65 1994. 616.1'20754–dc20. DNLM/DLC. 94–42060 CIP.

ISBN 978-3-211-82650-8

This book is dedicated to our children

Contents

Chapter 1

Introduction

"Everything should be as simple as can be, but not simpler."
Albert Einstein

The past decade has been marked by a trend from invasive to noninvasive intraoperative monitoring. As far as respiratory monitoring is concerned, initial experience with transcutaneous gas analysis laid the foundation for widespread clinical use of pulse oximetry and end-tidal gas analysis. It has been long recognized that echocardiography might become an equally useful adjunct to cardiovascular monitoring.

The fundamental purpose of cardiac monitoring is to warn the anesthesiologist of existing or impending cardiac abnormalities, so they can be corrected or prevented before the patient is harmed. Forces within and outside of medicine are pressuring our specialty to improve cardiovascular monitoring. For instance, the average age of the population is increasing, resulting in more elderly patients presenting for major surgical procedures. At the same time, the medical-legal establishment stands ready to hold anesthesiologists accountable for almost any adverse outcome associated with anesthesia or surgery.[1] In an effort to deal with this pressure, anesthesiologists have often resorted to invasive cardiovascular monitoring. However, invasive procedures are expensive, and even in the most experienced hands, they sometimes result in complications. In the past few years, with the development of modern computerized medical ultrasonics, anesthesiologists have recognized the usefulness of transesophageal echocardiography (TEE) as a new monitoring technique. TEE is the most complex, sophisticated, and potent cardiovascular monitor ever introduced. Although many applications of TEE are emerging, its three major uses in intraoperative monitoring are assessment of left ventricular preload and contractility, and detection of myocardial ischemia.[2]

Accurate estimates of left ventricular filling and ejection can be obtained by quantitative (off-line) assessment of TEE images. For instance, Harpole et al.[3] found a better correlation between echocardiographic and radionuclide estimates of end-diastolic volume and ejection fraction intraoperatively, than between pulmonary artery diastolic pressure and either radionuclide or echocardiographic estimates of the same variables. In practical terms, however, the quantitative analysis necessary is too time-consuming to be of value in the operating room. In contrast, qualitative (on-line) estimates of left ventricular filling and ejection are used in many leading anesthesia centers as a guide for the administration of fluids and inotropes.[4-6] Moreover, marked changes in filling and ejection can occur before, simultaneously with, or in the absence of changes in blood pressure or filling pressures. Cahalan[1] now uses TEE instead of pulmonary artery catheterization for intraoperative monitoring of patients in San Francisco. Even when both monitors are in place, they preferentially consult the TEE images in critical situations such as acute hypotension, because the information needed most (preload and contractility) is instantly apparent from TEE but not from the pulmonary artery tracing. Finally, the value of TEE has dramatically increased since it has been recognized that two-dimensional echocardiography is an earlier and more sensitive and specific marker of acute myocardial ischemia than traditional monitors.[7–10] Studies have not shown hemodynamics to be predictive of myocardial ischemia; most ischemia is noted during apparently normal hemodynamics.

Thus, TEE technique has now been well studied in anesthesia and intensive care unit (ICU) settings. As a continuous monitor that allows better evaluation of ventricular preload, ejection, and myocardial ischemia than other traditional monitoring methods, it has a potent impact on clinical management and decision making. TEE has enjoyed a substantial increase in use in the past few years (Fig. 1.1). This new technology has made anesthesiologists the natural users of TEE in the operating room. TEE, like pulmonary artery catheterization, is a technique that crosses interdisciplinary boundaries: it has piqued the interests of cardiologists, anesthesiologists, and cardiac surgeons. Unlike pulmonary artery catheterization, however, TEE equipment is much more expensive and requires specific technical, interpretative expertise and skill not readily available to all anesthesiologists.[11] Few anesthesiologists have a cardiology-echocardiography background, and they must learn the basics as they use the equipment. Formal guidelines for training anesthesiologists to use TEE have not been published. Certainly, it is generally felt that fellows in anesthesia should be provided with some formal training in TEE. Attempts are being made in the USA to resolve this issue by setting credentialing standards so that anesthesiologists can be certified to use and interpret TEE readings.[11,12] Until then, it

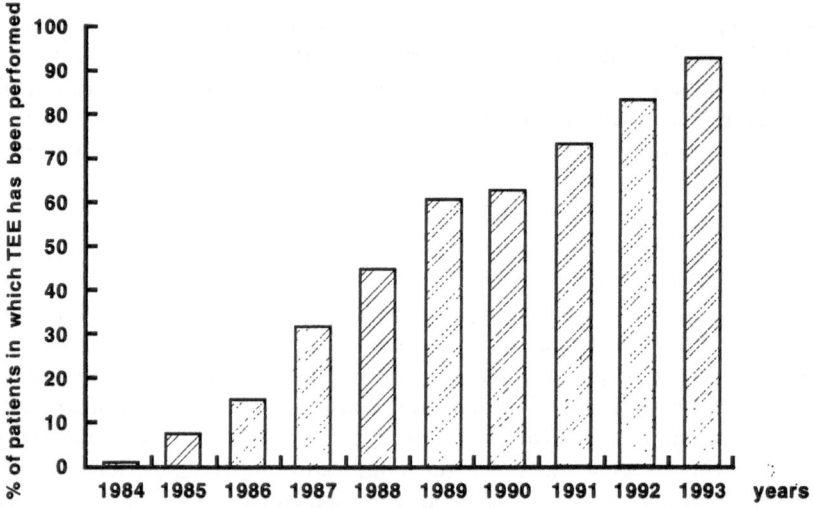

Fig. 1.1. Increase in the use of TEE in leading anesthesia centers in the USA. Sources: Simpson,[11] Rafferty et al.[15]

is advisable that interpretation be reviewed and confirmed by a trained cardiologist-echocardiographer.[11] Nevertheless, after some clinical training, the experienced anesthesiologist is able visually to assess ventricular global and regional function by relaying on the "educated eye". Furthermore, two-dimensional and Doppler echocardiography provides physiologic information for the quantitative assessment of ventricular function. An important role for anesthesiologists is to prove an objective interpretation of the effect of drugs, narcotic agents, and surgical intervention on ventricular function. In this regard, off-line analysis of echocardiography, as a research tool, can provide a more accurate physiologic approach to the assessment of ventricular performance.

Indications for intraoperative TEE monitoring are as follows[13]:

1. In primarily healthy patients, but where the operation is expected to compromise or deteriorate cardiac function (e.g., cross-clamping of the aorta or great vessels).
2. In patients with heart disease[14] (ASA class $\geqslant$ 3, Goldman index $\geqslant$ 12 points for intraoperative monitoring of left ventricular function in cardiac and non-cardiac surgical procedures.
3. As a diagnostic means in all unclear shock states, especially in acute circulatory insufficiency in the ICU as well as the operating room.
4. For fluid replacement in procedures in which large fluid shifts are expected (liver transplantation, septic states, etc.).
5. For controlled administration of vasoactive, inotropic, and diuretic drugs intraoperatively and in the ICU.

Contraindications to TEE: esophageal and gastroduodenal bleeding, as well as esophageal stricture.[15]

TEE has been available in the Department of Anesthesiology and General Intensive Care at the University Hospital of Vienna for more than six years and has been used primarily as a monitoring technique as described above (anesthesia indications for TEE). Therefore it seems appropriate to us to review our experience in order to clarify the value of this technique in the operating room and ICU for ourselves and others. The purpose of this book (based on our experience as well as our research interests) is to offer a comprehensive overview of all possible applications of TEE for evaluating ventricular function, mainly focusing on the monitoring capabilities of this fascinating technology. It is inevitable that the scope of the book prevents us from being able to cover all subjects of interest.

This book is intended primarily for those young anesthesiologists and colleagues in ICUs who are learning the technique of transesophageal echocardiography. It may also be of interest to cardiologists, internists, and radiologists who assess cardiac patients.

The experience reflected in this book is the result of joint work by anesthetists and cardiologist. We would like to express our thanks to Prof. C.K. Spiss, Prof. A. Hammerle, Prof. W. Haider, Prof. H.G. Kress, Prof. F. Lackner, Dr. G. Ihra, and many others who have been enthusiastic about the use of TEE in their everyday routine practice in our institution. We also acknowledge the valuable help of Mr. H.

Rinder from the Department of Anesthesiology for preparation of computer graphics and Dr. K. Leitner and Ing. P.A. Kunz, both from Firma Hewlett Packard, Vienna, Austria, who have collaborated in the preparation of the book. Finally, we also thank Faith McLellan, Director of the Manuscript and Grant Preparation Service of the Department of Anesthesiology, The University of Texas Medical Branch, Galveston, Texas, USA, for editorial review of this material. It is always a pleasure to work alongside Springer and the advice and assistance from this Company is greatly appreciated.

References

1. Cahalan MK. Non-invasive cardiovascular monitoring. 41st Annual Refresher Course Lectures, ASA, Las Vegas, p 411, 1990
2. Cahalan MK. Myocardial ischemia and performance. Anesth Clin North Am 9: 581–590, 1991
3. Harpole DH, Clements FM, Quill T, Wolfe WG, Jones RH, McCann RL. Right and left ventricular performance during and after abdominal aortic aneurysm repair. Ann Surg 209: 356–362, 1989
4. Kikura M, Shanevise JS, Levy JH. Intraoperative assessment of myocardial function. Curr Opin Anesth 7: 42–57, 1993
5. Reich DL, Konstand SN, Nejat M, Abrams HP, Buseck J. Intraoperative transesophageal echocardiography for the detection of cardiac preload changes induced by transfusion and phlebotomy in pediatric patients. Anesthesiology 79: 10–15, 1993
6. Leung JM, Levine E, Mangano MD. Intraoperative preload estimation using transesophageal echocardiography (Abstr). Anesthesiology 77: A125, 1992
7. Ellis JE, Shah MN, Briller JE, Roizen MF, Aronson S, Feinstein SB. A comparison of methods for detection of myocardial ischemia during noncardiac surgery: Automated ST-segment analysis system and transesophageal echocardiography. Anesth Analg 75: 764–772, 1992
8. Harris, SN, Gordon MA, Urban MK, O'Connor TZ, Barash PG. The pressure rate quotient is not an indicator of myocardial ischemia in humans. Anesthesiology 78: 242–250, 1993
9. Owall A, Ehrenberger J, Brodin LA. Myocardial ischemia as judged from transesophageal echocardiography and ECG in the early phase after coronary artery bypass surgery. Acta Anaesth Scand 37: 92–96, 1993
10. Voci P, Bilotta F, Aronson S, Scibilia G, Caretta Q, Mercanti C, Marino B, Thisted R, Roizen MF, Reale A. Echocardiographic analysis of dysfunctional and normal segments before and immediately after coronary bypass graft surgery. Anesth Analg 75: 213–218, 1992
11. Simpson JI. Anesthesia and the patient with co-existing heart disease. Little, Brown, Boston, p 61, 1993
12. Pearlman AS, Gardin JM, Martin RP. Guidelines for optimal physical training in echocardiography: Recommendation of the American Society of Echocardiography. Committee for Physician Training in Echocardiography. Am J Cardiol 60: 158–163, 1987
13. Heinrich H. Intraoperative echocardiography. In: Roelandt JRT, Sutherland GR, Iliceto S, Linker DT, eds. Cardiac Ultrasound. Churchill Livingstone, Edinburgh, pp 799–802, 1993
14. Wong T, Detsky AS. Perioperative cardiac risk assessment for patients having peripheral vascular surgery. Ann Int Med 116: 743–753, 1992
15. Rafferty T, LaMantia KR, Davis E, Phillips D, Harris S, Carter J, Ezekowitz M, McKloskey G, Godek H, Kraker P, Jaeger D, Kopriva C, Barash P. Quality assurance for intraoperative transesophageal monitoring: A case report of 846 procedures. Anesth Analg 76: 228–232, 1993

Chapter 2

General theory, history and development

Principles of two-dimensional echocardiography

Echocardiography (M-mode) was first described by Dr. Inge Edler (Fig. 2.1) working at the university of Lund, Sweden, in 1954. The term echocardiography refers to a group of tests that use ultrasound to examine the heart and record information in the form of echoes, i.e., reflected sonic waves.[1] The upper limit for audible sound is 20 KHz. The sonic frequency used for echocardiography ranges from 1 to 10 MHz (these are known as ultrasound waves). The characteristics of a sound wave can be expressed as a sine wave. The distance between two similar areas along the wave path (e.g., the distance that wave travels during a single cycle) is termed a wavelength (λ). The number of the wavelengths per unit time is the frequency (f) of the sound wave, which is measured in cycles per seconds (cps, also called Hertz [Hz]). One of the fundamental principles in sound physics is:

$$c = f\lambda \tag{1}$$

where c is the speed of sound in a medium, f is the frequency of the sound wave, and λ is the wavelength of the sound in the medium. The frequency of the sound depends only on the source that is producing it, but the speed of sound (and hence of wavelength) varies from one medium of propagation to another.[1]

The resolution of the recording, which is the ability to distinguish two objects that are spatially close together, varies directly with the frequency and inversely with the wavelength. The echocardiographic transducer provides two types of resolution, axial and lateral resolution. Axial resolution is the ability to differentiate between points lying along the path or axis of the beam, whereas lateral resolution refers to the ability to differentiate points lying in the plane perpendicular to the beam path.

Axial resolution of an ultrasonic beam is related to its wavelength or frequency and to the duration of the transmitted pulse. To illustrate the effects of wavelength and pulse duration on resolution, let us first calculate the wave lengths of two pulses of ultrasound: one of 2.5 MHz and second of 5 MHz. The first is most frequently used in adult transthoracic echocardiography and the second in transesophageal echo-cardiography. According to the formula (1) and the fact that the speed of the sound in tissue is approximately 1500 m/sec, therefore, for the first case,

$$f = 2,500,000 \text{ Hz}$$

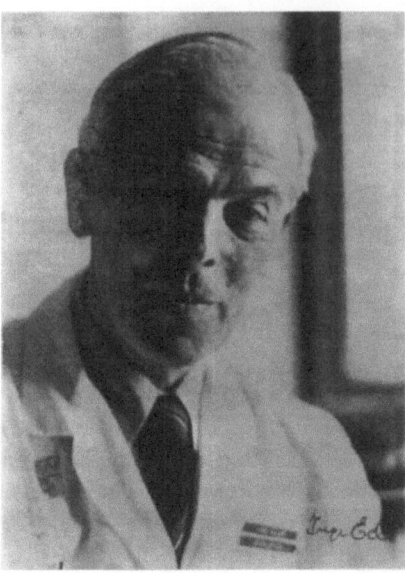

Fig. 2.1. Dr. Inge Edler, the first to demonstrate the potential of ultrasound for cardiac diagnosis (1954). For his pioneering work he is generally recognized as "the father of echocardiography"

$$\lambda = \frac{1,500 \text{ m/sec}}{2,500,000 \text{ cps}}$$

$$\lambda = 0.0006 \text{ m or } 0.6 \text{ mm}$$

for the second case,

$$f = 5,000,000 \text{ Hz}$$

$$\lambda = \frac{1,500 \text{ m/sec}}{5,000,000 \text{ cps}}$$

$$\lambda = 0.0003 \text{ m or } 0.3 \text{ mm}$$

The wavelength of 2.5 MHz pulse, therefore is 0.6 mm, whereas the 5 MHz pulse is 0.3 mm.

Assume that a sound pulse of 4 cycles is transmitted into a test medium (Fig. 2.2) in which two objects (O_1 and O_2) are located at 6.2 and 6.3 cm from the transducer. At lower frequency (2.5 MHz), the total length of the sound pulse is 2.4 mm ($\lambda = 0.6$ mm × 4 cycles = 2.4 mm). With a pulse train of this length, the echo from the closer of the two objects (O_1) is still striking the transducer when the echo from the second object (O_2) returns. The echocardiograph, therefore, senses and displays one long echo rather than two discrete echoes representing each of the reflecting surfaces. In contrast, when a frequency of 5 MHz is used, the wavelength is 0.3 mm. With the same 4-cycle pulse train, the total pulse length is only 1.2 mm ($\lambda = 0.3$ mm × 4 = 1.2 mm). At this pulse duration, there is a relatively long interval between the

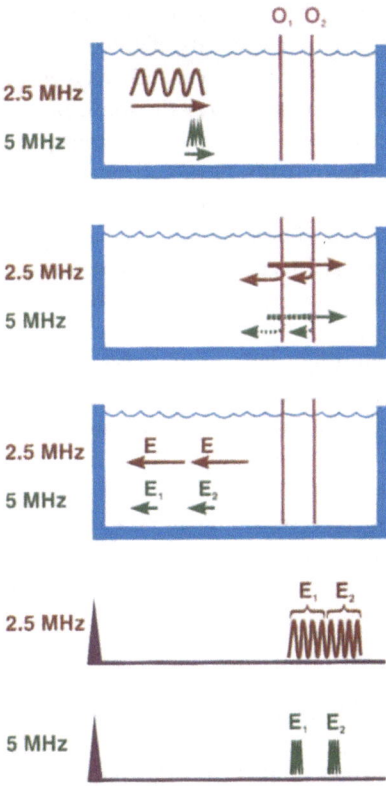

Fig. 2.2. The effects of frequency on axial resolution. In the upper panel, two pulses of four cycles each, one from a 2.5 MHz transducer, and one from a 5 MHz transducer, are emitted into a medium. Because of the higher frequency, the pulse from the 5 MHz transducer is shorter than the corresponding pulse from the lower-frequency transducer. When these pulses strike two objects O_1 and O_2, echoes are reflected at both interfaces. Because the shorter pulse duration at a higher frequency (5 MHz) separate reflections (O_1 and O_2) arise from each object and are recorded as distinct. At the lower frequency (2.5 MHz), the pulse length is such that the echoes from O_1 and O_2 are continuous, and hence, these objects cannot be "resolved" as separate

return of the echo from the first object and that from the second object. Thus, two separate echoes are displayed by the echocardiograph, and the presence of two distinct reflecting interfaces is "resolved". The example shows that high-frequency (short wavelength) ultrasound can identify separate object that are less than 1–2 mm apart. Beams having lower frequency (longer wavelength) have poor resolution. However, the degree of penetration, which is the ability to transmit sufficient ultrasonic energy into the chest and/or to provide satisfactory recording, is inversely proportional to the frequency of the signal.[2] Since a high-frequency ultrasonic beam (i.e., 5 or 8 MHz) is unable to penetrate a thick chest wall, lower frequency ultrasonic beams are used in adult transthoracic echocardiography (2.5–3 MHz) and higher

(5 MHz) in transesophageal echocardiography. For this reason transesophageal echocardiography provides a better quality of images than transthoracic approaches.

Piezoelectric crystals are the transmitters and receivers of the ultrasonic waves used in echocardiography. These crystals form the main part of the transducer (probe). Typically, the piezoelectric crystals send intermittent pulses of sound at 2.5–5 MHz and receive the reflected signal. When the ultrasound beam strikes an interface of different densities, for example, that between the endocardium and blood, a portion of the ultrasound is reflected. These signals, when amplified and processed, can be imaged on a television screen. Electronic circuits measure the time delay between the transmitted and received signals. Using the known speed of ultrasound in tissue, the time delay is converted into a precise distance measurement from transducer to tissue.

By rapid, repetitive scanning (with multiple crystals in phased array, series) along many different radii within an area in the shape of a sector (fan, arc), echocardiography generates a two-dimensional image of an anatomic section of the heart. Thus, two-dimensional image are formed by sweeping multiple, individual beams across 80° to 90° of arc. The time needed for performing an entire sweep of the sector arc is sufficiently short, so that the resulting image is considered a still frame of a moving object. The two-dimensional scan is repeated 30 to 60 times per second. The human eye and brain are quite adept at assimilating these rapidly generated images, which create the illusion of continuous motion, "live" (real time) images of the interrogated anatomic section of the heart.

The core of any echo system is a timer (Fig. 2.3). It sends a synchronization signal to the probe and to the oscilloscope. The piezoelectric transducer converts the electric impulse into an ultrasound, which is transmitted into the medium. After the transmission of the short sound pulse, the same probe is used for reception. The time lag between the start pulse and the received echo will be proportional to the distance between the probe and the reflecting structure. As a result, the reflecting structure is seen at the corresponding depth.

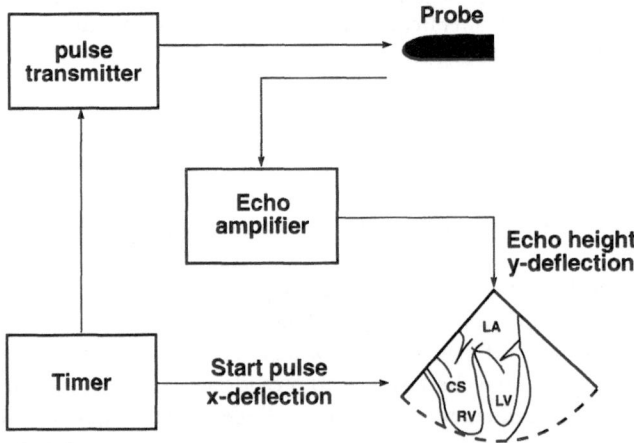

Fig. 2.3. Block diagram of an echo apparatus showing its major components

The scattering of sound energy in all directions as the transmission pulse proceeds, as well as progressive loss of amplitude (attenuation), reduces the energy available for echoes coming from greater depths. For compensation of this loss and improving the quality of the two-dimensional image, there are a variety of controls that modify the echocardiogram. These controls can greatly influence the echo display and, as will be demonstrated, are vitally important in the recording of specific cardiac echoes. Beginning with the examination the echocardiographer must make important stepwise selections and adjustments.

— The first step is appropriate adjustment of *transmit control*, which aligns the entire image.
— The second step is *compression*, which sets up a gray scale. Gray scale indicates the ability of a display to record both bright and weak echoes in varying shades of gray.

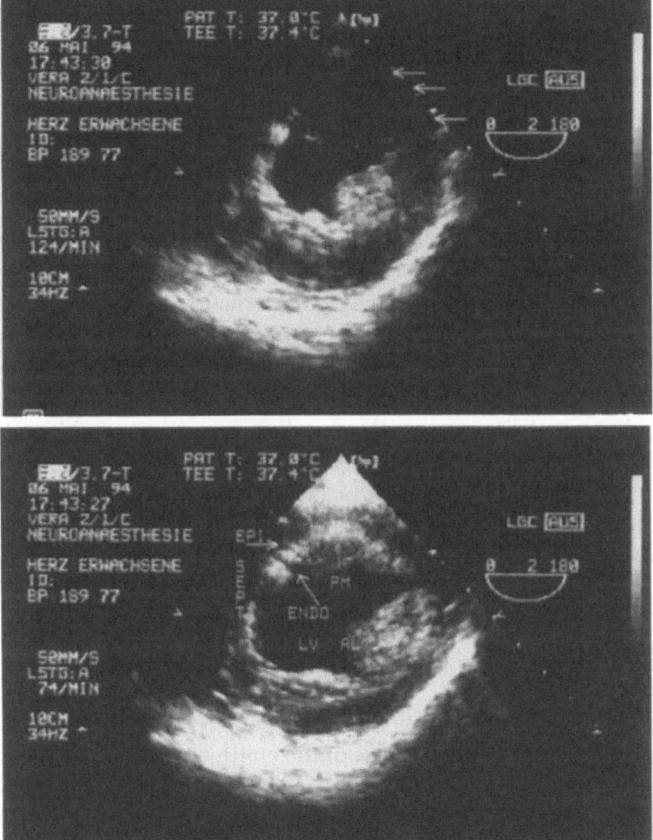

Fig. 2.4. Top: Left ventricular short axis cross-section of the left ventricle with low-gain area shown by arrows. Bottom: The same area after higher optimal gain. The posterior part of the left ventricular wall with endo- and epicardium can now be appreciated

— The third step represents *time gain compensation* (TGC) or "depth compensation." TGC controls affect the alignment of the image at specific horizontal levels (regions). These regions corresponds to the location of the TGC lever on the system's control and compensate for the natural loss in echo intensity or strength that occurs as the beam penetrated more deeply. To achieve this ends, the TGC consists of an amplification circuit, which selectively increases the strength of far-field echoes, as well as a ramp function, which permits individual control of the level and the rate at which this depth-dependent amplification is brought into play. By varying the slope of this ramp, one can rapidly employ full amplification at a particular level or can cranially increase amplification as a function of time or depth. The TGC control is undoubtedly the most confusing and frequently the most difficult control for the echocardiographer to use.[2] If one remembers that the purpose of this device is to compensate for the loss of ultrasonic energy or attenuation as the beam enters the body structures, then one better understands how the control should be used. The anesthetist in the routine practice of monitoring with the two-dimensional mode (preload, cardiac output, and regional wall motion) is primarily interested in endo- and epicardial borders. How critically visualization of these structures depends on the gain control is illustrated in Fig. 2.4.

Principles of Doppler echocardiography

Modern ultrasonographs can measure the Doppler shift while simultaneously producing two-dimensional echocardiograms. The Doppler principle or shift, as defined by Christian Johann Doppler, Vienna, Austria, in 1842 (Fig. 2.5), states that any apparent shift in transmitted frequency occurs as a result of motion of either the source or the target. The classic example is the change in pitch of a train whistle as the train approaches and then passes the observer (Fig. 2.6). In cardiology, the source of the sound (ultrasound) is the transducer and the target is the red blood cells moving in the heart and great vessels. When the ultrasound beam strikes a moving object, the reflected sound returns to the transducer with a slightly altered frequency. The frequency shift detected by the Doppler mode is directly related to the velocity at which the red blood cells are travelling within the ultrasound beam and the cosine of the angle (θ) at which the red cells are insonated by the stationary transducer, i.e.,

$$V = \frac{c}{2f_0} \times \frac{\Delta f}{\cos \theta}$$

In this formula V equals the velocity of blood flow, Δf equals the Doppler frequency shift (which is measured) or difference of the emitted and reflected signals, f_0 equals the frequency of the emitted ultrasound signals, c equals the velocity of sound in tissue (approximately 1540 m/sec), and θ equals the angle of incidence between the direction of blood flow and the direction of the emitted ultrasonic signal. Modern ultrasound machines directly compute velocity from frequency shift.

The Doppler recording is a spectral display (towards the transducer, positive, and away from the transducer, negative). Thus, spectral analysis of the Doppler shift

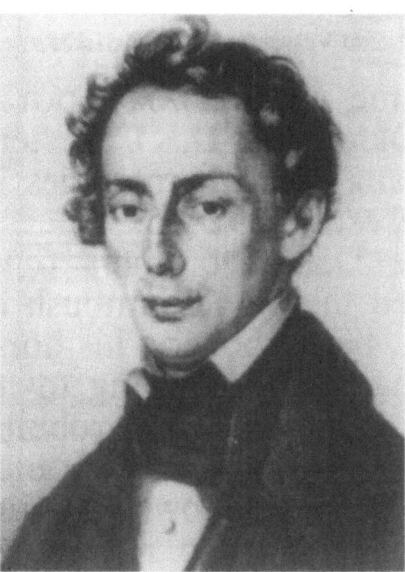

Fig. 2.5. Christian Johann Doppler, Austrian mathematician and physicist who first enunciated the principle that perceived frequency of traveling wave is altered by motion of the source or the receiver (1842), and this effect has subsequently borne his name

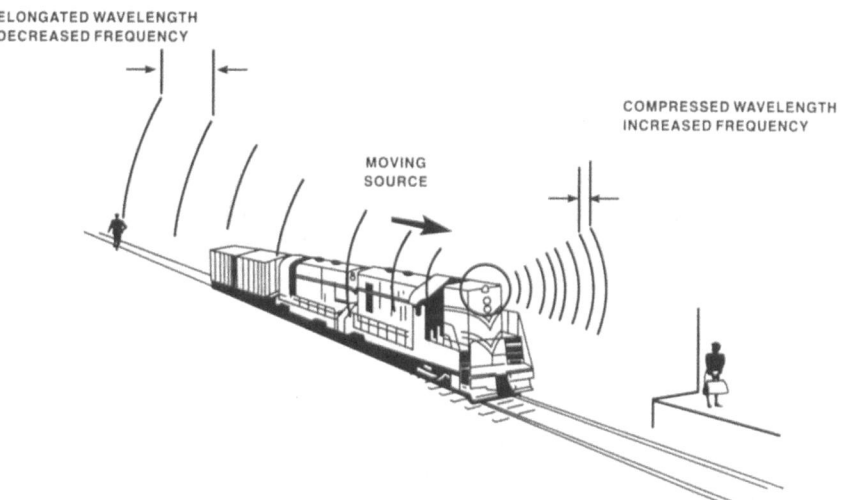

Fig. 2.6. As the train moves toward the observer, the wavelengths are compressed, and the frequency of the sound waves, or pitch, is perceived as being increased. Likewise, as the train moves away from the receiver, the wavelengths are elongated and the frequency of the waves, or pitch, is perceived as being decreased

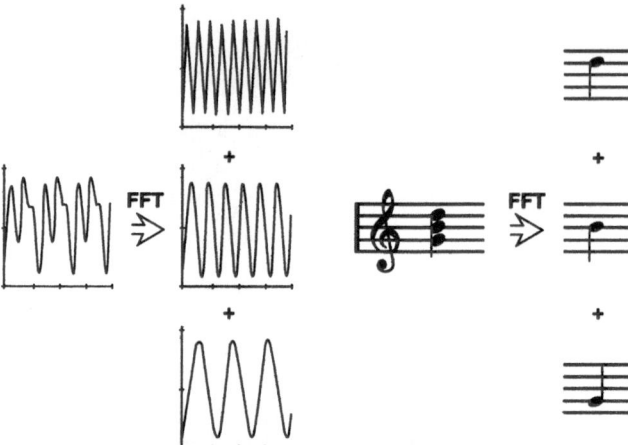

Fig. 2.7. The FFT (fast Fourier transformation) isolates the individual frequencies present in the complex wave containing Doppler frequency shift information

provides a graphic display of blood flow velocities plotted over time. Because all blood cells do not move at the same velocity, they will create a variety of frequency shifts. These shifts return to the transducer as a complex wave that contains information about the motion of all blood cells moving at a variety of velocities within the ultrasound beam. This complex signal is then processed through a computer that does a calculation called an FFT (Fast Fourier Transformation). An analogy for this FFT process is the differentiation of the individual notes present in a musical chord (Fig. 2.7).

It should be pointed out that the angle between the transducer and the flow direction plays a major role in quantitations. If the flow and the sound beam are parallel (in the Doppler equation, the angle of incidence is $\cos 0° = 1$), the velocity can be calculated without correction of the angle.[3–5] In contrast, by real time two-dimensional images for more backscattered sound energy, the optimal angle between the ultrasound beam and the interrogated surface is 90°. Hence, we can detect left ventricular endo- and epicardial surfaces best in short-axis cross-sectional view, but left ventricular Doppler transmitral inflow for evaluation of ventricular diastolic function requires a four-chamber view or with omniplane probe transgastric view at 90°.[6,7] Similarly, measurement of Doppler cardiac output by TEE sampling of the aortic or pulmonic valves can be performed appropriately only when the direction of the ultrasound beam and the interrogated blood flow are nearly parallel.[8,9]

With respect to the measurement of blood flow rate by Doppler ultrasound it should be noted that there are two different data acquisition modalities:

The first one is continuous wave Doppler, which can measure any high velocities (such as occurs in severe valvular stenosis) from within the heart and accurately display them on a monitor. Although continuous wave Doppler can record high velocities it is not capable, because of the manner in which the information is obtained, of determining where the signal originated because all frequency shifts

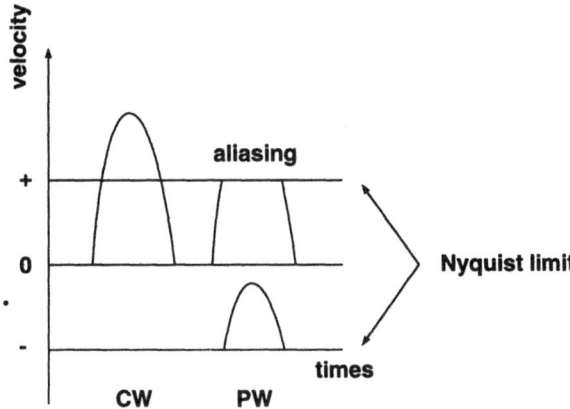

Fig. 2.8. Schematic representation of Nyquist limit by pulsed Doppler wave. *CW* continuous wave; *PW* pulsed wave

detected along the path of the Doppler beam will be incorporated in a final signal display. Thus, continuous wave Doppler has range ambiguity as its main drawback.

The second modality is pulsed wave Doppler, which is almost the direct opposite of the continuous wave modality in both its advantages and disadvantages. It can measure the blood flow at a specific depth and ignore ultrasonic reflections from other flows intercepted by the beam. Because of the possibility of aliasing, pulsed Doppler limits the maximum measurable Doppler frequency shift (Nyquist limit) and hence blood flow velocity. When the Nyquist limit is exceeded, ambiguity occurs (i.e., aliasing phenomenon) in the interpretation of any velocity information displayed (Fig. 2.8). The trade-off for the ability to measure flow at precise locations is that ambiguous velocity information is obtained when flow velocity is high. A simple reference to movies about the American West clearly illustrates this point. When a stagecoach gets underway, its wheel spokes are observed as rotating in the correct direction. As soon as a certain speed is attained, however, rotation in the reverse direction is noted. This reversal occurs because the camera film rate is too slow to correctly observe the motion of the wheel spokes. In pulsed Doppler, the ambiguity exists because the measured frequency shift and the sampling frequency are in the same frequency range. Ambiguity is avoided only if the Doppler frequency shift is less than half the sampling frequency. The aliasing effect is the major drawback of the use of the pulsed Doppler. Practically, the continuous wave mode has superiority over pulsed Doppler only when high blood flow velocities (such as those that occur as a result of the formation of jets) must be estimated.

Color Doppler images can be considered simply as a combination of pulsed wave Doppler and two-dimensional echocardiography. In a conventional pulsed Doppler modality, velocities are typically displayed in spectral form from a single sample volume of interest. By using multigated Doppler, multiple sample volumes can be placed along a line of interest, as is shown in Fig. 2.9. Returned signals are electronically converted to a color spectral scale and by means of a computer are superimposed on the simultaneously acquired two-dimensional images. The direction

Pulsed Doppler   **Color Doppler**

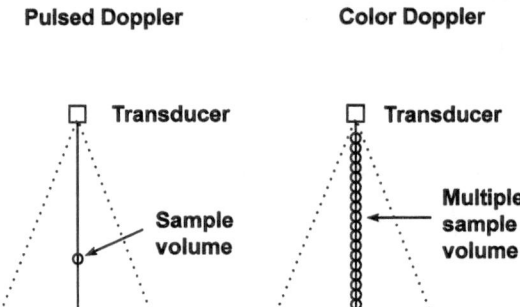

Fig. 2.9. Pulsed Doppler and color Doppler sample volume. At any given time, the measurements obtained using pulsed Doppler are assessed only in a small area called the sample volume. This sample volume must be placed in the expected area of flow on the two-dimensional image. Color Doppler generates the same type of flow information, but produces a "moving" color picture of the flow occurring in the heart by the ultrasonic beam's investigation of a large number of sample volumes along successive transmission beams

of the blood flow is displayed in color: usually blood flow away from the transducer is blue, and flow towards the transducer is red. The viewer is presented with an instantaneous, albeit quantitative, image of intracardiac blood flow. The Nyquist limit (aliasing) for color Doppler corresponds to that for conventional pulsed wave Doppler.

Doppler echocardiography is gaining widespread use and is rapidly becoming an important tool for anesthesia practice. Aside from the well-established utility of Doppler echocardiography in cardiology for diagnosing valvular lesions and shunts, its application in the assessment of ventricular function is undergoing active clinical investigation. The important feature of this utility is that with Doppler echocardiography both systolic and diastolic function can be estimated:

— ventricular systolic function by means of semilunar (aortic, pulmonalis) Doppler outflow measurements,
— ventricular diastolic function by means of transmitral and transtricuspidal Doppler inflow measurements.

The Bernoulli equation and measurement of the Doppler peak velocity of a tricuspid regurgitant jet offer another avenue for the estimation of right ventricular systolic pressure.[10] Tricuspid regurgitation is a common finding with Doppler echocardiography, even in normal subjects. If an optimal signal is not obtained by Doppler alone, signal enhancement can be obtained by simultaneous injection of saline. The peak velocity of the tricuspid regugitant jet (V) reflects the pressure difference between the right ventricle and the right atrium. According to the Bernoulli equation:[10]

$$\Delta P = 4 \times V^2$$

where ΔP is the pressure gradient (in millimeters mercury) and V is the instantaneous regurgitant jet velocity (in meters per second).

Addition of the tricuspid gradient to the mean right atrial pressure provides right ventricular systolic pressure. (Mean right atrial pressure can be estimated by measuring jugular venous pressure and converting it to mm Hg, or an empirical value of 5, 10, or 15 mm Hg, based on the size of the right atrium, can be used as the mean right atrial pressure). In the absence of pulmonary stenosis (which is very rare), this derived figure for right ventricular systolic pressure should be equal to pulmonary artery systolic pressure. Further extrapolation of this technique may be applied to the noninvasive estimation of the pulmonary artery diastolic pressure. If pulmonic regurgitation is present (not rare), the end-diastolic velocity of the pulmonic regurgitation jet can be used to calculate the gradient between the pulmonary artery and right ventricle at end-diastole. When added to the mean right atrial pressure, this gradient may provide the pulmonary arterial diastolic pressure.

Digital cine loop technology

Cine loop analysis is a recent development that allows the acquisition of echocardiographic images in a digital form as a sequence of a determined frame number, starting from a trigger signal, normally the R wave of the QRS peak of the simultaneously recorded electrocardiogram. This technique makes it possible to collect predetermined echocardiographic images (frames) in a digital form during a single cardiac cycle. These images, once obtained, can be reviewed in a cyclic manner, i.e., *cine loop*, and in a particular screen format, usually the quad screen format (Fig. 2.10) or dual screen

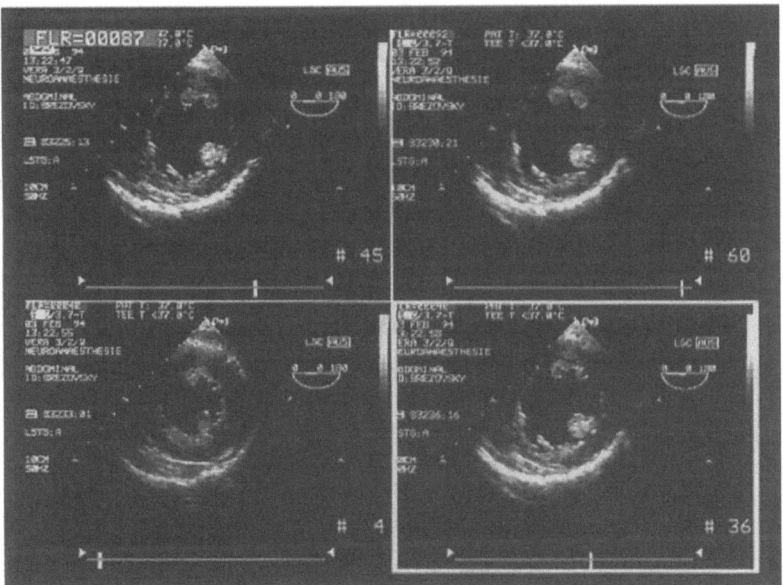

Fig. 2.10. Quad screen format cine loop

format, so that loops acquired at differing times during the investigation can be compared in synchrony with the cardiac cycle.[11] Thus, it is possible to compare the instant wall motion pattern with the baseline pattern. This system greatly enhances the possibility of detecting differences and changes without the disturbing interference of visual memory pitfalls.

The image source for cine loop analysis is usually the video signal produced by the echocardiographic machine or a videotape recorder. To produce a correct synchronization of acquired images between different cardiac cycles, a signal of physiological meaning, as a trigger for the acquisition start, is required. The R wave of the QRS complex is a universal marker for the beginning of systole; and the echocardiograph can easily recognize the R wave and use it for its triggering function. During the examination period the electrocardiogram must be without artifact (electrode problems, motion of the patient, etc.). The image acquisition effectively starts when the operator presses the corresponding key and the first trigger signal has been recognized.

The most important part of the system is the cine loop video memory. Memory size is the paramount determinant of the maximal quality of images stored for elaboration. Each single image represents a frame.[12] In other words, a frame is the whole image information that the monitor screen can visualize. Current memories contain 30 or more frames. This number depends on the modality of the division of the screen and on the image resolution (pixel density). The screen area can be divided into halves (dual or split screen), or three or four (quad screen) regions with source images. As image loops can be independently acquired in each single portion of the screen, the maximum number of stored images is given by the maximum single frame number multiplied by the regions represented in each single screen. The acquired image is reduced so as to fit the screen region occupied. The video memory can also be divided into blocks: 32, 16, 12 or 8 consecutive frames. Every sequence of n consecutive frames ($n = 8, 12, 16, 32$) constitutes "a loop." The maximum number of acquired loops is given by the maximum frame number divided by the frame number in each single loop (Fig. 2.11). The possible numbers are: 4 loops by 8 frames, 3 loops by 12 frames, 2 loops by 16 frames, 1 loop by 32 frames. Each frame is identified by a specific progressive number (#1–32). The technical expression for this concept is "dynamic video memory." The time interval between two consecutive frames (interimage delay) can be selected by the software. Each loop will cover a total interval of[13]:

$$(n-1)* \text{ interimage delay,}$$

where n = number of frames per loop. A 50-msec interimage delay in an 8-frame loop will cover a total of 350 msec. Since there is currently great interest among anesthesiologists in detecting visually qualitative segmental wall motion abnormalities, this interval permits the acquisition of the whole cardiac cycle in a wide range of heart rates. The acquired series of images is displayed on the computer monitor in a cyclic manner, the first frame immediately after the last one. A play-loop delay-setting-operation can speed up or reduce the motion velocity.

The amazing feature of digital cine loop technology is the possibility of acquiring images from the same portion of the cardiac cycle from different times during the

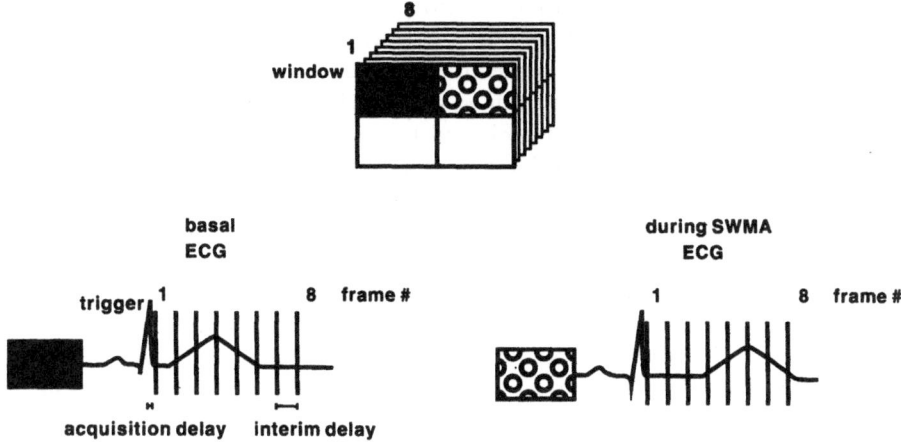

Fig. 2.11. The digital cine loop system can acquire images using the R wave of the electrocardiographic tracing as a trigger signal. It is possible to choose an acquisition and an interimage (interim) interval. At each interval a single frame is captured and stored in a digital memory. The video memory is divided into 8 frames, which constitute a "loop." When there is a difference in heart rate between the basal status and observation the two cardiac cycles can be played synchronously. In this example, the cardiac cycle should be divided into 8 consecutive parts or interimages, starting from a triggering R wave of the ECG until the next R wave.
SWMA segmental wall motion abnormality

investigation and simultaneously reviewing them (Fig. 2.10) side by side on the screen. To make sense from a physiological point of view the loops must be representative of the same part of the cardiac cycle.[14] If the heart rates are different, they can be synchronized using the same interim delay (Fig. 2.11). Baseline images, intermediate images and the image at the moment of observation can be compared. For the time being, the clinical use of cine loop technology in anesthesia is mainly segmental wall motion analysis for the detection of ischemia. The operator can easily and correctly evaluate changes in wall motion without relying on memory.[13]

History and development of transesophageal echocardiography

Transesophageal echocardiography was introduced by Frazin et al.[15] in 1976, a short time after the clinical acceptance of echocardiography. The original TEE transducer was a single crystal (M-mode) in a lozengelike housing suspended from a wire. They studied awake patients who were able to swallow this device. They showed that conventional M-mode measurements could be made that closely agreed with those recorded by precordial echo using changes in left ventricular volume to monitor its function. Later, Matsumoto et al.[16] applied a similar M-mode probe to the intra-operative monitoring of left ventricular dimensions in patients undergoing open heart surgery. Of special importance among their observations was the finding that the surgical freeing of the heàrt from its restraint by mediastinal strictures and the pericardium was accompanied by a delayed inward motion of the septum.

In 1981, Mitsuztaki et al.[17] reported the detection and localization of myocardial infarction by M-mode TEE. In twenty patients with coronary artery disease, they found good agreement between TEE and left ventriculography in classifying the severity of anteroseptal wall motion abnormalities. Nevertheless, this work did not attract the attention of anesthesiologists because of the lack of spatial orientation in M-mode. In 1982, with the introduction of a two-dimensional echocardiographic transducer by Schulter et al.[18] (Germany), which could be positioned in the esophagus, intraoperative echocardiography became a practical tool for anesthesiologists. Over the next four years, a number of publications demonstrated the feasibility and potency of this technique.[19] However, anesthesia interest in this technique remained limited, as the image quality was poor and only morphological information could be obtained. It was not until the introduction of the second generation of single (transverse) plane transesophageal probes in 1986–87 that the combination of high-resolution imaging (5 MHz) and color flow was provided.[20] The good resolution of images attracted the attention of many anesthesiologists and lead to fundamental investigations concerning the intraoperative use of the TEE as an invaluable monitoring tool in patients at risk for acute ischemia.[21,22]

Characteristics of transesophageal systems

All transesophageal transducers have basically the same construction. They essentially consist of an ultrasound transducer mounted at the tip of a flexible endoscope that has a maximum shaft diameter of 10 to 11 mm, and a total shaft length of 70 to 120 cm. The guidance control allows the tip at least 90° of anteroposterior flexion and up to 70° of lateral mobility in each direction (Fig. 2.12A). These mobilities are effected mechanically by two wheels on the endoscope handle with the possibility of locking the steering controls. Most current generation probes use an operating frequency around 5 MHz and are comprised of a phased-array transducer containing 48–64 elements. The ultrasound elements are mounted at the distal flexible tip so as to provide *transverse* plane images of the heart, i.e., their scan plane is at an angle 90° to the shaft of the endoscope.

Recently, biplane and omniplane or multiplane transesophageal probes have been constructed in an attempt to overcome the lack of versatility associated with imaging structures only in the transverse plane. *Multiple examination* with an omniplane probe from a single transesophageal location by a rotatable transducer (Fig. 2.12B) was conceived almost a decade ago and constituted the next logical step in imaging options. It has only recently been realized from Hewlett Packard (Fig. 2.13). This system allows free rotation of the imaging plane from 0° or transverse (perpendicular to the endoscope's long axis), to 90°, or longitudinal (parallel to the endoscope's long axis), and further to 180° (transverse with left-right inversion).[23,24] Thus, the sectors of the obtainable planes encompass a cone, with the tip originating in the transducer. Plane rotation is effected by automated control buttons in the echoscope handle. The angle between current and transverse (or 0° plane) is shown on a external dial on a screen. The probe has capabilities for pulsed, continuous wave and color Doppler

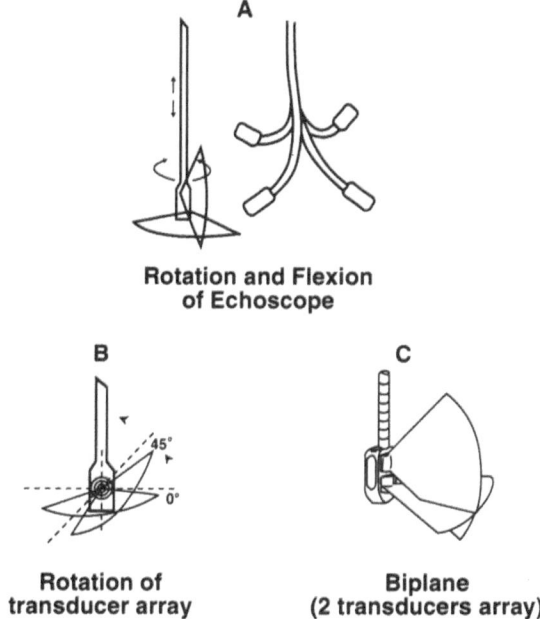

Fig. 2.12. Schematic representation of transesophageal imaging plane possibilities that are determined from the movements of the transducer array. (A) Rotation and flexion of the standard echoscope. (B) Additional intermediary planes by rotation of the transducer phased array. (C) Biplane or two-transducer phased array

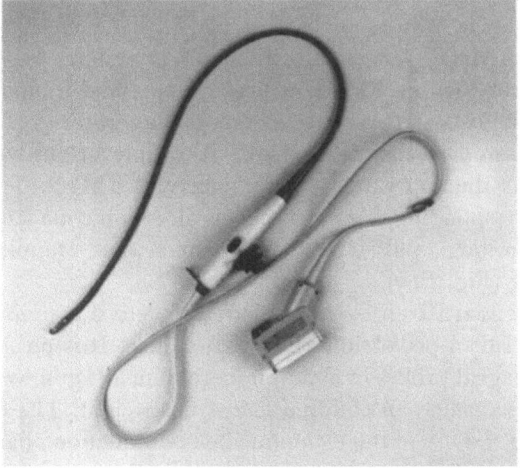

Fig. 2.13. Commercially available multiplane (omniplane) Hewlett Packard transesophageal probe

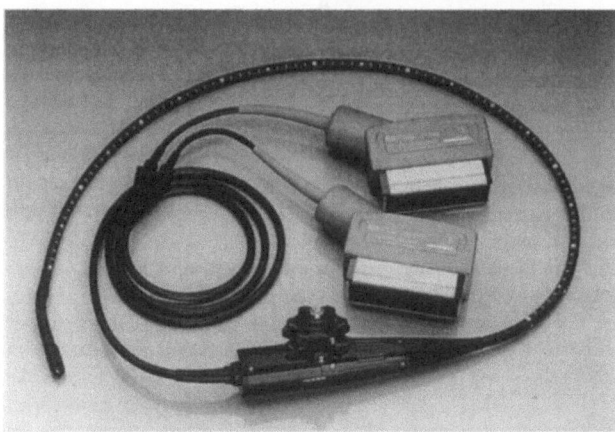

Fig. 2.14. Commercially available biplane Hewlett Packard transesophageal probe

imaging. Multiplane devices achieve intermediate plane orientations more easily than biplane (see below) instruments and may be considered the best currently available technology.

Alternatively, biplane transesophageal probes [Hewlett Packard, Andover, MA; (Fig. 2.14) also Aloka, Tokyo and Corometrics, Wallingford, CT] consist of two phased-array transducers mounted side by side; one imaging in transverse and the other in longitudinal plane, Fig. 2.12C). The distance between the centers of the two transducers is approximately 1 cm. With this probe, transverse and longitudinal scanning can be performed in an alternating fashion, but not simultaneously. Because of the finite separation between the two elements, slight repositioning of the probe may be necessary to image precisely the same segment of tissue.

Other manufacturers of transesophageal probes include Acuson (Mountain View, CA), which makes a transesophageal probe with 64 elements that operates at a frequency of 5.0 MHz. General Electric Medical Systems (Milwaukee, WI) offers a single-plane probe with a 64 elements transducer and a biplane probe with two 64-element transducers. Advanced Technology Laboratories (ATL, Bellevue, WA; Toshiba, Japan; and Diasonics, Palo Alto, CA) supply a transesophageal echo probe with 64 elements that operates at a frequency of 5 MHz. The TEE probes are interfaced to corresponding standard echocardiographic machines, providing combined two-dimensional, pulsed, and continuous wave Doppler, as well as color Doppler imaging (Fig. 2.15).

The size of standard transesophageal transducers is a serious limitation to the application of TEE in pediatric anesthesia practice. It is possible to use standard adult transesophageal probes in children more than 20 kg in weight, but only small probes can be used safely in children below this weight. The current size of TEE probes also limits the use of the technique before induction of anesthesia and in the postoperative period for prolonged monitoring, both representing high-risk periods for the development of ischemia in patients with coronary artery disease. Thus, technological effort should be directed towards the further miniaturization of

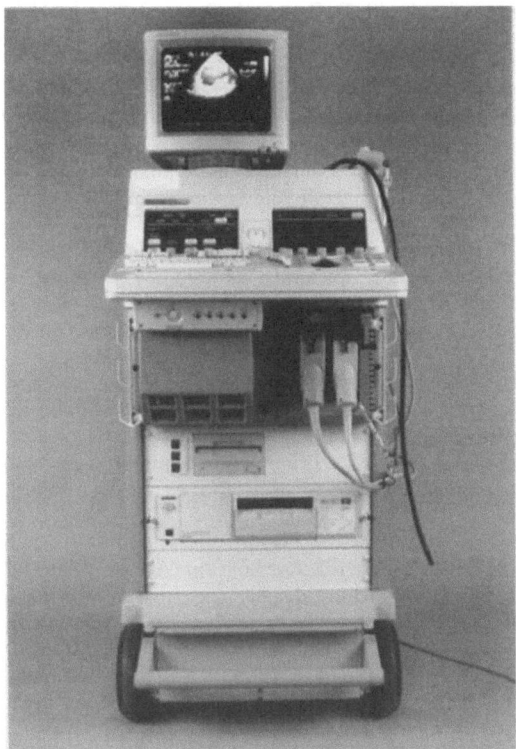

Fig. 2.15. Commercially available new Hewlett Packard ultrasonograph *Sonos* 2500 suitable for intraoperative TEE investigation

the phased array elements and the provision of higher frequencies for improved resolution.

Safety considerations: Both trauma (cuts and bites) and chemical agents used in cleaning the probe can cause deterioration and breaks in the coating of the insulating material. Such breaks may not be apparent on simple visual inspection. Thus, manufacturers' recommendations for both cleaning and sterilizing the probe and checking it regularly for electrical leakage must be adhered to rigorously. Alcohol should not be applied to the tip of the probe because it penetrates the rubber seals and damages the transducer.

References

1. Carlsen EN. Ultrasound physics for physicians: A brief review. J Clin Ultrasound 3:69–74, 1975
2. Feigenbaum H. Echocardiography. 5th ed. Lea & Febiger, Philadelphia, 1994
3. Sahn DJ. Instrumentation and physical factors related to visualization of stenotic and regurgitant jets using Doppler echocardiography. J Am Coll Cardiol 12: 1354–1358, 1988

4. Saini VD, Nanda NC, Maulik D. Basic principles of ultrasound and Doppler effect. In: Nanda NC, ed. Doppler echocardiography. 2nd ed. Lea & Febiger, Philadelphia, London, pp 3–24, 1993

5. Kolev N. Assessment of left ventricular function in ischemic heart disease using pulsed Doppler transmitral blood flow during exercise. J Cardiovasc Diag Proc (NY) 11: 15–18, 1990

6. de Bruyne B, Lerch R, Meier B, Schlaepfer H, Gabathuler J, Rutischauser W. Doppler assessment of left ventricular diastolic filling during brief coronary occlusion. Am Heart J 117: 629–634, 1989

7. Huemer G, Kolev N, Kurz A, Zimpfer M. Influence of positive end-expiratory pressure on left and right ventricular performance assessed by Doppler two-dimensional echo-cardiography. Chest 106: 67–73, 1994

8. Katz WE, Gasior TA, Quinlan JJ, Gorcsan J. Transgastric continuous wave Doppler to determine cardiac output. Am J Cardiol 71: 853–857, 1993

9. Darmon PL, Hiller Z, Mogtader A, Mindich B, Thys D. Cardiac output by trans-esophageal echocardiography using continuous wave Doppler across the aortic valve. Anesthesiology 80: 796–805, 1994

10. Saini VD, Nanda NC, Maulik D. Principles of Doppler ultrasound implementation. In: Nanda NC, ed. Doppler echocardiography. 2nd ed. Lea & Febiger, Philadelphia, pp 18–23, 1993

11. West SR, Feigenbaum H, Armstrong WF, Green D, Dillon JC. Split screen simultaneous digital imaging of rest and stress echocardiogram (Abstr). J Am Coll Cardiol 3: 563, 1984

12. Feigenbaum H. Digital recording, display and storage of echocardiograms. J Am Soc Echocardiogr 1: 378–382, 1988

13. Marganelli V, D'Ambrosio G, Carella L, Iliseto S, Rizzon P. A digital cine loop technology—a new tool for the evaluation of wall motion abnormalities. In: Iliseto S, Rizzon, Roelandt JRTC, eds. Ultrasound in coronary artery disease. Kluwer Academic Publ, Dordrechts, pp 95–99, 1991

14. Iliseto S, Sorino M, D'Ambrosio G, Papa A, Biasco G, Rizzon P. Detection of coronary artery disease by two-dimensional echocardiography and transesophageal atrial pacing. J Am Coll Cardiol 5: 1188–1197, 1985

15. Frazin L, Talano JV, Stephanidis L. Esophageal echocardiography. Circulation 54: 102–108, 1976

16. Matsumoto M, Oka Y, Srom J. Application of transesophageal echocardiography to continuous intraoperative monitoring of left ventricular performance. Am J Cardiol 46: 95–99, 1980

17. Matsuzaki M, Matsuda Y, Yoshinoby I. Esophageal echocardiographic left ventricular anterolateral wall motion in normal subjects and in patients with coronary artery disease. Circulation 63: 1085–1091, 1981

18. Schulter M, Langenstein BA, Polster BA. Transesophageal cross-sectional echocardio-graphy with a phased array transducer system. Technique and initial clinical results. Br Heart J 48: 67–71, 1982

19. Hanrath P, Kremer P, Langenstein BA, Matsumoto B. Detection of ostium secundum atrial septal defects by transesophageal cross-sectional echocardiography. Br Heart J 49: 350–355, 1983

20. Chapman JV, Vandenbogaerde J, Everaert JA, Angelson BAJ. The initial clinical evaluation of a transesophageal system with pulsed Doppler, continuous wave Doppler, and color flow imaging based on an array technology. Int J Cardiac Imaging 5: 9–16, 1989

21. Abel MD, Nishimura RA, Callahan MG, Rehder K, Ilstrup DM, Tajik J. Evaluation of intraoperative transesophageal two-dimensional echocardiography. Anesthesiology 66: 64–68, 1987

22. Clements FM, de Bruijn NP. Perioperative evaluation of regional wall motion by transesophageal two-dimensional echocardiography. Anesth Analg 66: 249–261, 1987

23. Flachkampf FA, Hoffmann R, Verlande M, Schneider W, Ameling W, Hanrath P. Initial experience with multiplane transesophageal echotransducer: assessment of diagnostic potential. Eur J Cardiol 13: 1201–1206, 1992
24. Kolev N, Ihra G, Leitner K, Spiss CK, Zimpfer M. Improved detection of perioperative myocardial ischemia with multiplane (Hewlett Packard) transesophageal scanning: Two-dimensional biplane and transmitral Doppler echocardiography. J Cardiovasc Diag Proc (NY) (in press) 1994

Chapter 3

Standard transesophageal imaging and planes

General considerations

After induction of anesthesia and intubation of the patient's trachea, the TEE probe can be inserted. By lifting the mandible together with the tongue with one hand, the probe can then be introduced with other hand. For successful introduction, it is important to direct the tip of the probe towards the midline of the pharynx. The depth of anesthesia must be adequate to prevent undesirable reactions to the stress of the introduction of the probe, which is, at worst, comparable to the stress produced by tracheal intubation. Before introduction, the tip of the probe should be lubricated, and the steering controls of the probe should be unlocked so that it can gently follow the contours of the pharynx. In cases where blind introduction of the probe is difficult, direct visualization of the proximal esophagus with the laryngoscope is helpful. The technique is almost identical to tracheal intubation and therefore should be easy for an anesthetist to handle. As there is a potential risk of causing esophageal damage (or even perforation) force should never be used when introducing the probe. Similarly, the probe should not be advanced or withdrawn while the tip is flexed or retroflexed or in the locked position.

Cardiac examination

A comprehensive TEE examination entails a sequence of transducer positions and anatomic planes of sections. A step-by-step approach is suggested that can be altered on the basis of the clinical situation. Detailed reviews of imaging orientations and anatomic correlations of the tomographic sections of the heart have been published.[1,2] The three standard transverse views are illustrated in Fig. 3.1. During TEE examinations using a biplane or multiplane (omniplane) probe, sequential views of the transverse and longitudinal planes can be obtained. Table 3.1 summarizes the various standard biplane TEE views which are most used in anesthesia and ICU.

Transgastric views

The probe is advanced into the esophagus until the stomach is reached (between 38 and 42 cm from the incisors). Passage of the tip of the probe beyond the

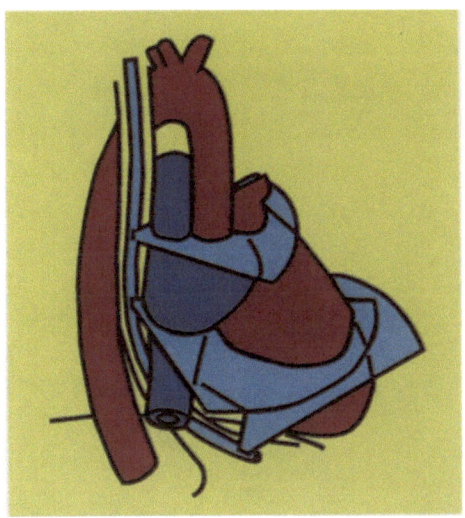

Fig. 3.1. Stylized representation of the heart, great vessels and esophagus, with the positions of the TEE probe from which the three basic series of transverse imaging planes are obtained

Table 3.1. Transverse plane and longitudinal plane views most used in anesthesia and ICU

Cardiac examination	Transverse plane	Longitudinal plane
Transgastric views (38–42 cm)	1. LV short-axis at level of papillary muscles 2. LV short-axis at level of mitral valve	1. LV transgastric long-axis view 2. transgastric LVOT view
Midesophageal views (29–33 cm)	1. LV four-chamber view 2. LV five-chamber view 3. coronary sinus and RV inflow	1. LV two-chamber view
Basal views (25–28 cm)	1. short-axis of the RVOT, PA and aortic valve 2. coronary arteries	long-axis view of ascending aorta or PA

LV left ventricle; *LVOT* left ventricular outflow tract; *RV* right ventricle; *RVOT* right ventricular outflow tract; *PA* pulmonary artery.

gastroesophageal junction is recognized by the appearance of echoes from the liver. Anticlockwise rotation usually brings the heart into view, and the tip should be anteflexed and withdrawn to obtain transverse short-axis tomographic views of the heart at the level of the papillary muscles (Figs. 3.2 and 3.3) and mitral valve. The left ventricle is displayed to the reviewer's right and the interventricular septum to the viewer's left. Posterior structures are viewed at the top of the video screen and the anterior structures at the bottom. Transgastric left ventricular short-axis views are used to assess and monitor ventricular filling, regional wall motion abnormalities and global left ventricular function.[3–6]

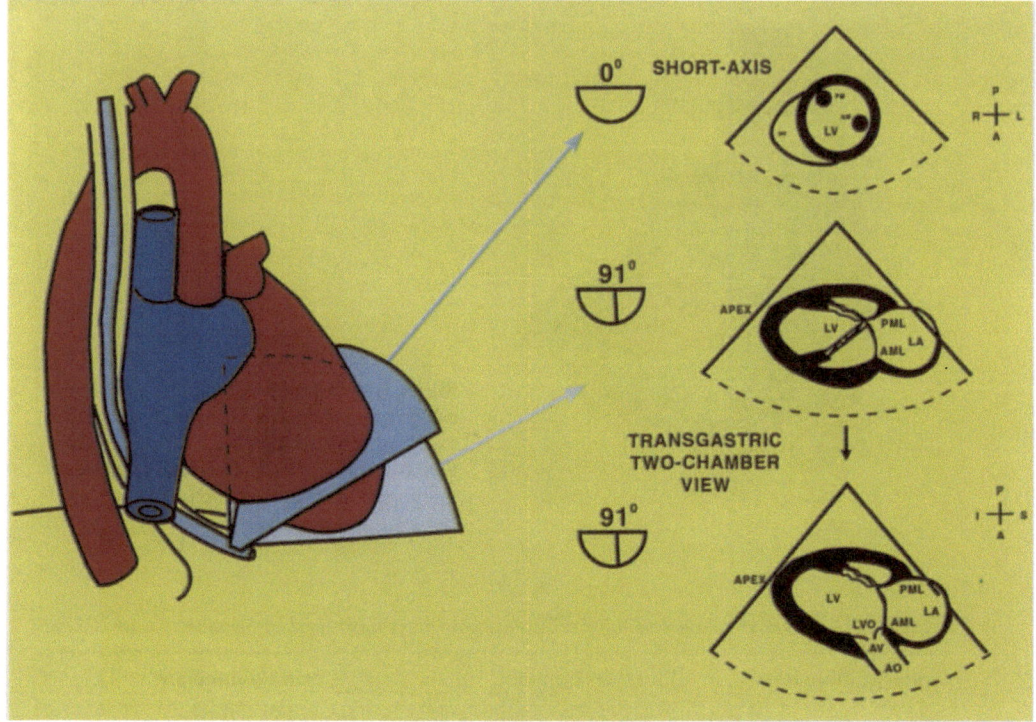

Fig. 3.2. Schematic diagram illustrates the left ventricular short-axis cross-section and long-axis from the transgastric position using omniplane or biplane transesophageal probe. *AML* anterior mitral leaflet; *AO* aorta; *AV* aortic valve; *LA* left atrium; *LV* left ventricle; *LVO* left ventricular outflow tract; *PL* anterolateral papillary muscle; *PM* posteromedial papillary muscle; *PML* posterior mitral leaflet; *RV* right ventricle; *P* posterior; *A* anterior; *R* right; *L* left; *S* superior; *I* inferior

By means of control buttons on the multiplane echoscope, rotation of the transverse scanning position from 0° to 90°, or by means of longitudinal scanning plane probe (biplane probe) permit a transgastric long-axis view (or transgastric longitudinal two-chamber view) of the left ventricle to be obtained (Figs. 3.2 and 3.4). Transgastric left ventricular long-axis view resembles an upside-down parasternal long-axis except that the left ventricular structures, including the true apex, are better visualized, while the left atrium and aortic valve are not well seen. The posterior left ventricular wall is displayed at the top of the video screen, the anterior wall at the bottom, the apex to the left, and the left atrium to the viewer's right. This view is good for assessment of apical and basal wall motion abnormalities.[7,8]

For optimal long-axis orientation, slight leftward or rightward flexion and rotation of the tip of the echoscope may be necessary. Further slight anteflexion of the tip (and some time slightly insertion of the probe) produces an apical long-axis equivalent view of the left ventricle and aortic and mitral valve (Figs. 3.2 and 3.5).

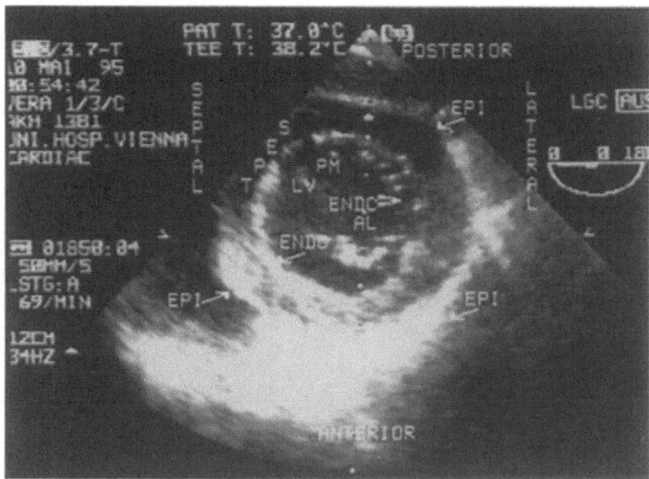

Fig. 3.3. TEE left ventricular short-axis cross-section of the left ventricle (standard monitoring position in anesthesia). *AL* anterolateral papillary muscle; *ENDO* endocardium; *EPI* epicardium; *LV* left ventricle; *PM* posteromedial papillary muscle; *SEPT* septum

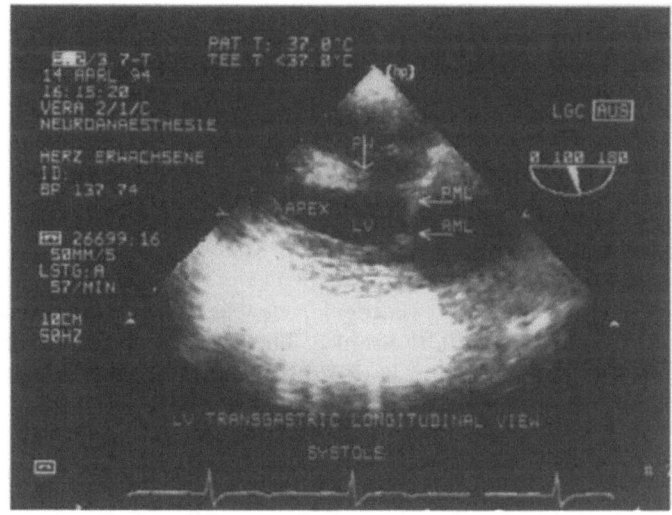

Fig. 3.4. Left ventricular transgastric longitudinal view obtained with omiplane TEE probe, achieved by rotating the scanning position in short-axis view from 0° to 90°. This view resembles an upside-down parasternal long-axis with visualization of the apex. *LV* left ventricle; *PW* posterior wall; *PML* posterior mitral leaflet; *AML* anterior mitral leaflet

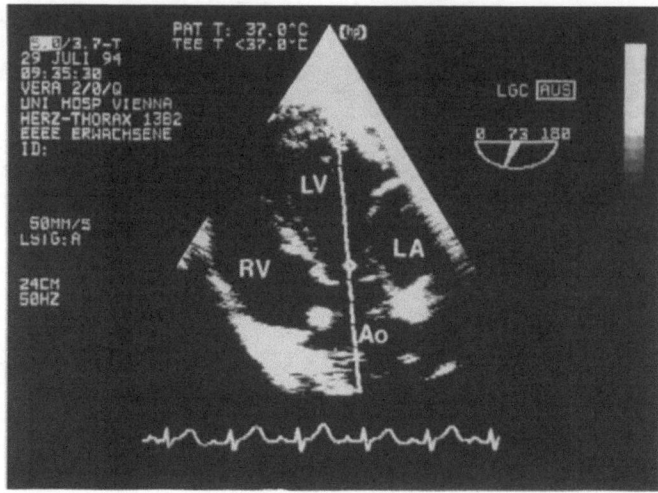

Fig. 3.5. Transgastric imaging of left ventricular outflow tract for estimation of Doppler left ventricular cardiac output by sampling the aortic valve. *Ao* aorta; *LA* left atrium; *LV* Left ventricle; *RV* right ventricle

This plane permits alignment of the Doppler beam parallel with the blood flow across the aortic valve and allows determination of left ventricular cardiac output or assessment of aortic valvular lesions.

Midesophageal views

The scope should be withdrawn slowly while maintaining contact with the anterior esophagus, and at approximately 29–33 cm from the incisors, tomographic four-chamber views of the heart are obtained by gently releasing anteflexion. Slight retroflexion of the probe tip is frequently required to obtain these views. From this transverse plane assessment of both atria, both ventricles and both atrioventricular valves can be accomplished (Figs. 3.6, 3.7). Much of the skill involved in performing a good and comprehensive right ventricular view lies in the subtle manipulation of the probe over the relatively short distance. The four-chamber views are dysplayed with the apex oriented downward. Both atria are on the top, the left ventricle to the viewer's right, and the right ventricle to the viewer's left on the video screen. It should be pointed out that in this plane the left ventricular apex is occasionally not well imaged. When the apex is visualized, it can be difficult to establish that the image is unassociated with an oblique angle of interrogation. A foreshortened image would significantly underestimate the left ventricular dimensions.[9]

From the four-chamber recording position, progressive anteflexion of the tip will display the left ventricular outflow tract and the long axis of the aortic valve and aorta (Fig. 3.8 left), similar to the transthoracic apical five-chamber view. Slight advancement and extreme retroflexion of the tip from the four-chamber recording

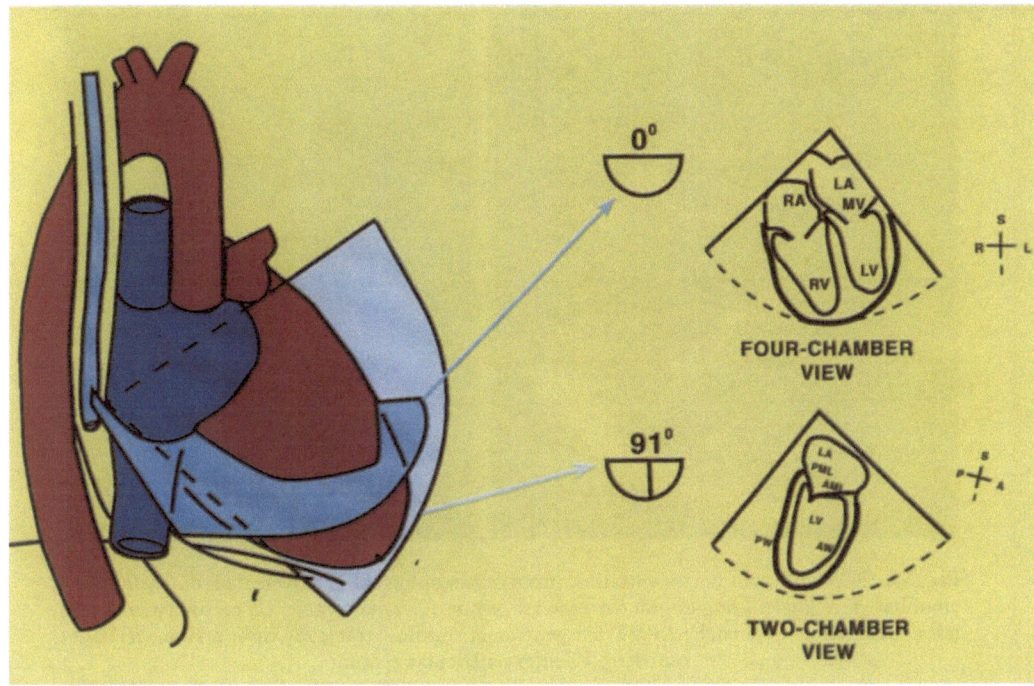

Fig. 3.6. Schematic diagram illustrating the midesophageal transverse and longitudinal scanning of the left ventricle. *AML* anterior mitral leaflet; *AW* anterior wall; *LA* left atrium; *LV* left ventricle; *MV* mitral valve; *PW* posterior wall; *RA* right atrium; *RV* right ventricle; *A* anterior; *P* posterior; *S* superior; *I* inferior; *R* right; *L* Left

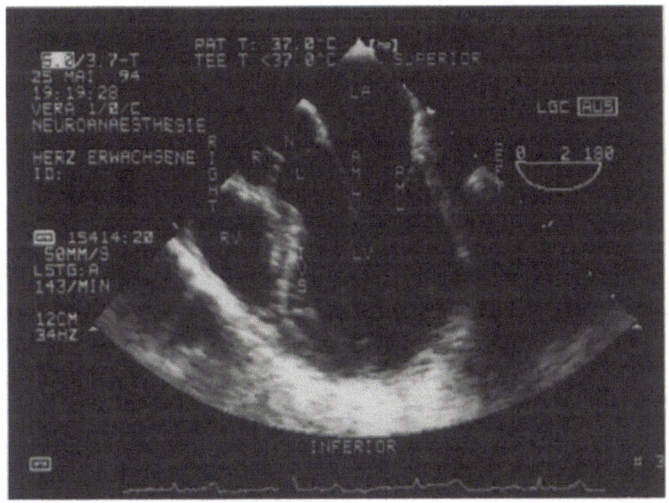

Fig. 3.7. Midesophageal transverse four-chamber view. *LV* left ventricle; *RV* right ventricle; *LA* left atrium; *RA* right atrium; *AML* anterior mitral leaflet; *PML* posterior mitral leaflet; *IVS* interventricular septum

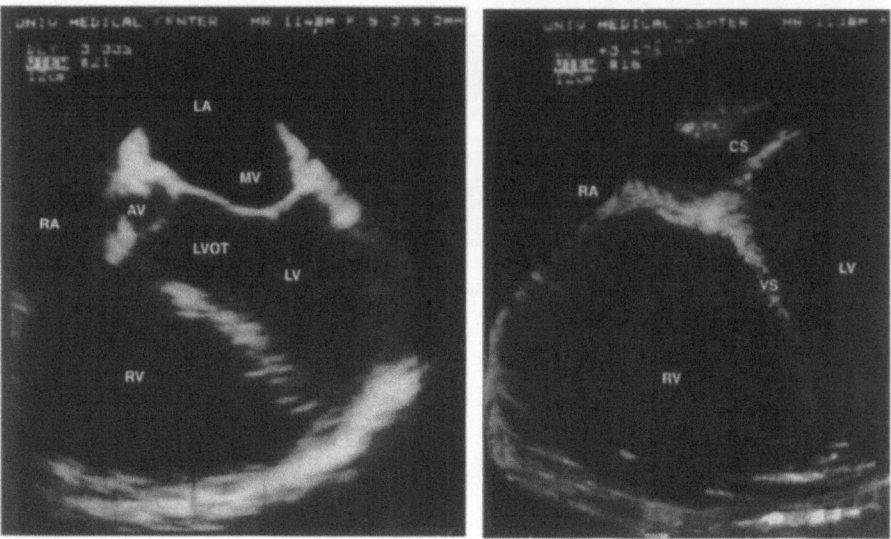

Fig. 3.8. Two different views obtained from midesophageal transverse plane. *Left*: Five-chamber view. *Right*: Long axis of the coronary sinus. *AV* aortic valve; *CS* coronary sinus; *LA* left atrium; *LV* left ventricle; *LVOT* left ventricular outflow tract; *RA* right atrium; *RV* right ventricle; *VS* interventricular septum

position will display the inflow tract of the right ventricle and long axis of the coronary sinus (Fig. 3.8 right). Midesophageal transverse tomographic sections from the various four-chamber planes allow assessment of the biventricular function, atriovnticular valves with their support structures, both atria, interatrial septum, interventricular septum and left ventricular outflow tract.[10,11]

From midesophageal transverse position, by means of control buttons on the multi-plane echoscope, rotation of the scanning position from 0 to 90°, or by means of longitudinal scanning probe (biplane probe) permit assessment of the left ventricular longitudinal two-chamber view. This section transects the left atrium, mitral valve orifice and left ventricle (Fig. 3.6). Midesophageal left ventricular longitudinal two-chamber view displays the left ventricular posterior wall to the viewer's left, the left ventricular anterior wall to the viewer's right, the left atrium to the top, and the left ventricular apex at the bottom of the video screen (Fig. 3.9 left). This view is very good for assessment of left ventricular apical wall motion abnormalities.[12]

Basal esophageal views

Progressive withdrawal and anteflexion of the probe at approximately 25–28 cm allows the examination of basal structures of the heart (Fig. 3.10). All transverse short axis-views displayed the anterior structures at the bottom of the video screen,

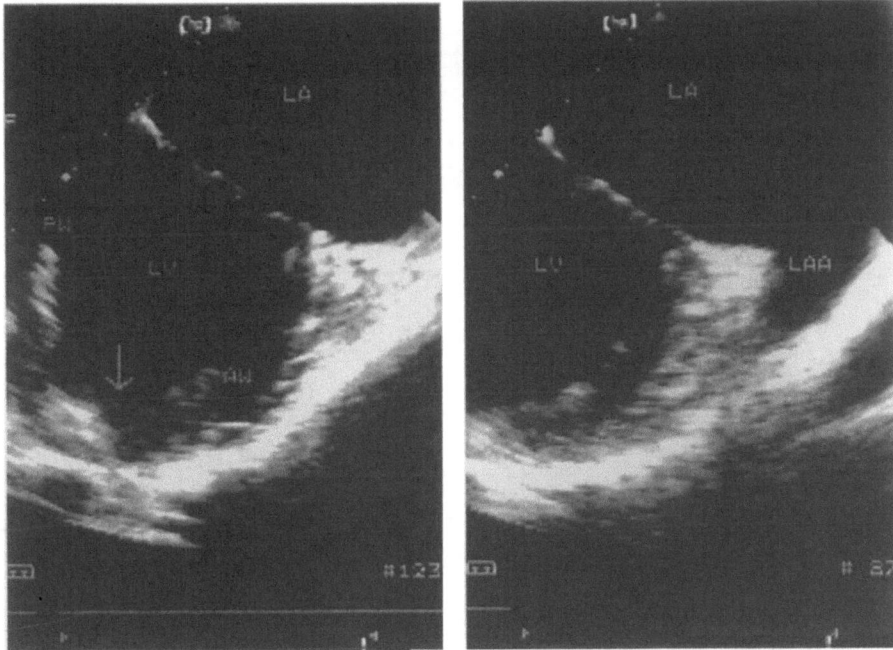

Fig. 3.9. Midesophageal longitudinal two-chamber view. *Left*: The arrow points to the left ventricular apex. *Right*: Slight clockwise rotation of the probe brings the left atrial appendage. *AW* anterior wall; *LA* left atrium; *LAA* left atrial appendage; *LV* left ventricle; *PW* posterior wall

posterior structures at the top, and left sided structures on the viewer's right. Tilting the tips superiority or by very slightly withdrawing the transducer produces sequential basal short axis scans. Basal short-axis scans sequentially depict the aortic valve, proximal ascending aorta, proximal coronary arteries, atrial appendage, superior vena cava, pulmonary veins and proximal pulmonary arteries. In this plane the visualization of the right ventricular outflow tract with pulmonic valve is optimal for Doppler assessment of cardiac output (Fig. 3.11).

The aortic valve cusps are usually imaged in the transverse short-axis plane. The aortic root is also very good seen in this view. The origin of the left main coronary artery and its bifurcation can be seen with an upward tilt of the tip of the transducer (Figs. 3.10 and 3.12 left). The right coronary artery is somewhat difficult to image and can usually be seen at a different tomographic level, with superior or inferior tilting of the tip of the transducer (Figs. 3.10 and 3.12 right).

Gradual withdrawal of the probe from the basal position allows examination of the ascending thoracic aorta up to 3 to 4 cm from the sinobulbar junction. Rotation of the probe to 90° permits investigation of the ascending aorta in longitudinal plane and further rotation until 180° reveals thoracic aorta in transverse plane.

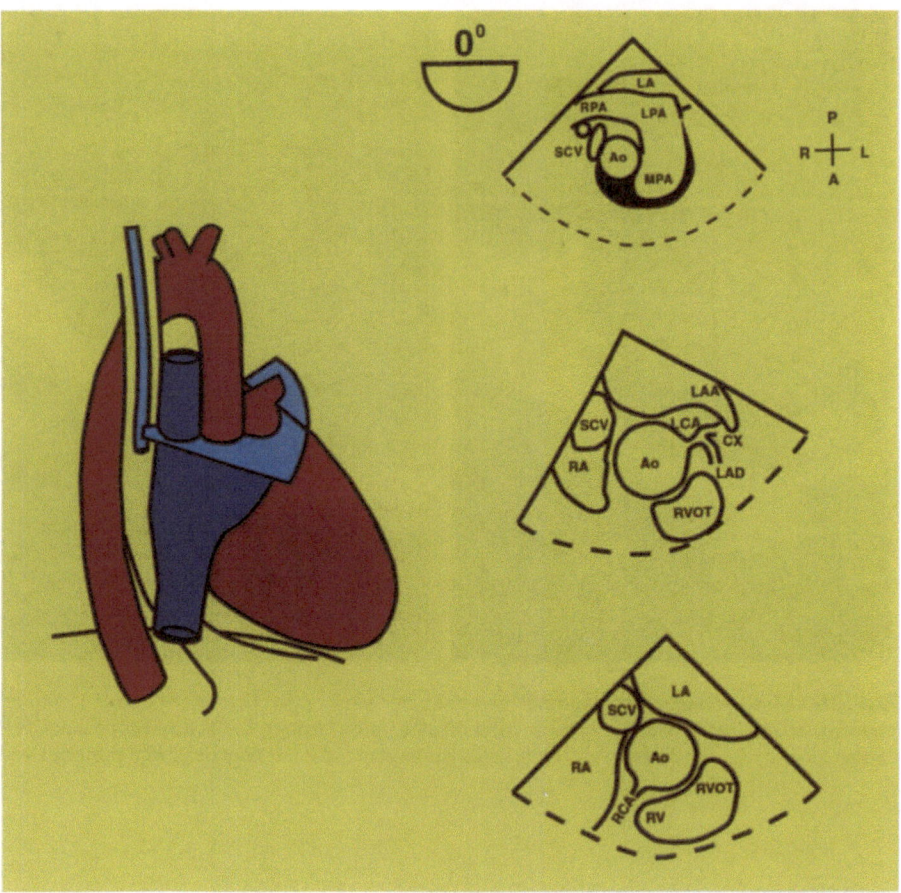

Fig. 3.10. Schematic diagram illustrating basal esophageal scanning of the pulmonary artery; aorta; and coronary arteries in the three different transverse planes. *Ao* aorta; *CX* circumflex coronary artery; *LA* left atrium; *LAA* left atrial appendage; *LAD* left anterior descending coronary artery; *LCA* main left coronary artery; *LPA* left pulmonary artery; *MPA* main pulmonary artery; *RA* right atrium; *RCA* right coronary artery; *RPA* right pulmonary artery; *RV* right ventricle; *RVOT* right ventricular outflow tract; *SCV* superior caval vein. *P* posterior; *A* anterior; *R* right; *L* left

In conclusion, because of time constrains and very narrow diagnostic goals the anesthesiologist performs a much more limited examinations than described in echo-cardiographic literature.[12] However, for complete monitoring an absolute minimum of three cross-sectional views should be attempted with a single-plane transducer and three additional views with a multiplane or biplane transducer (Table 3.2). Without these views correct interpretation of subsequent hemodynamic alterations during heart monitoring may be impossible.

Intraoperative TEE has proven to be a safe procedure.[13] Possible complications are transient vocal cord paresis,[14] probably as a result of abnormal sustained pressure on the laryngeal nerves and pharyngeal abrasion.

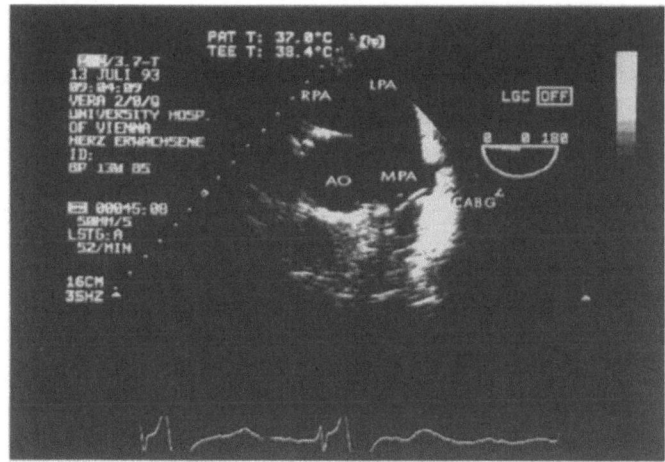

Fig. 3.11. TEE image of the pulmonic valve and main pulmonary artery by Doppler estimation of right ventricular cardiac output. *AO* aorta; *CABG* coronary artery bypass graft; *LPA* Left pulmonray artery; *MPA* main pulmonary artery; *RPA* right pulmonary artery

Table 3.2. The three main cross-sectional views which must be monitored with a single plane transducer and three additional views with multiplane or biplane transducer

Cross-section	Position of the trans-ducer in esophagus (depth from incisorsin cm)	Transducer or angle	Principal use
Pulmonary valve	basal (25–28)	transverse 0–10°	estimation of Doppler RV output
LV four-chamber transverse	midesophageal (29–33)	transverse 0°	monitor biventricular systolic and Doppler diastolic function
LV two-chamber long-axis	midesophageal (29–33)	longitudinal 80–100°	detect LV apical and basal SWMA
LV midpapillary short-axis	transgastric (38–42)	transverse 0–10°	monitor LV filling and SWMA
Transgastric LV long-axis	transgastric (38–42)	longitudinal 80–100°	detect LV apical and basal SWMA
LVOT and aortic valve	transgastric (39–42)	longitudinal 70–90°	estimation of Doppler LV output

LV left ventricle; *LVOT* left ventricular outflow tract; *RV* right ventricle; *SWMA* segmental wall motion abnormalities.

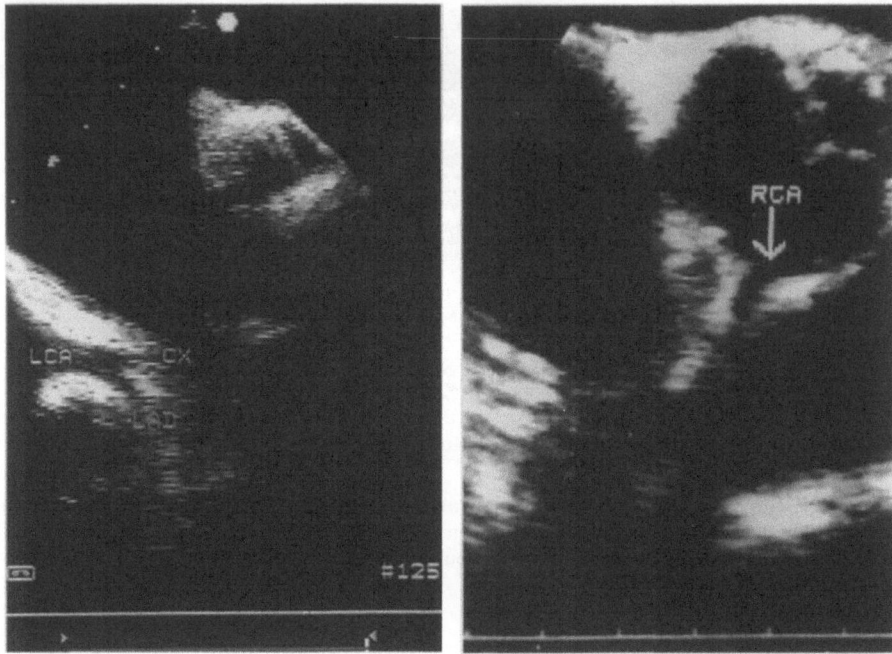

Fig. 3.12. Two basal transverse short-axis views of the coronary arteries. Left: The main left coronary artery (*LCA*) is imaged just above the left aortic cusp. Bifurcation into circumflex artery (*CX*) and left anterior descending coronary artery (*LAD*) is shown. Right: Right coronary artery (*RCA*) is given in another transverse section

Future development in transducer technology will include fixed and rotatable matrix transducers in which elements are arranged and electronically steered in a way permitting to center two orthogonal planes around the central beam,[14] thus, avoiding the offset between the two element sets, and allowing simultaneous (in real-time) image acquisition in both plane.

References

1. Fraser AG, Anderson RH. The normal examination: technique, imaging planes, and anatomical features. In: Sutherlandt GR, Roeland JRT, Fraser AG, Anderson RH, eds. Transesophageal echocardiography. Gower Med Publ, London, pp 3.1–3.26, 1991
2. Chandrasekaran K, Brown B, Bansal RC, Davis G, Karalis DG, Ren J. Transesophageal pulsed and color Doppler echocardiography. In: Nanda NC, ed. Doppler echocardiography. Lea & Febiger, Philadelphia, pp 175–198, 1993
3. Kikura M, Shanewise JS, Levy JH. Intraoperative assessment of myocardial function. Curr Opin Anesth 7: 42–52, 1993
4. Missri J. Transesophageal echocardiography. Clinical and intraoperative use. Churchill Livingstone, New York, Edinburgh, pp 19–40, 1993
5. Cahalan MK. Intraoperative monitoring for myocardial ischemia with two-dimensional transesophageal echocardiography. Anesth Clin North Am 9: 581–590, 1991

6. Harris SN, Gordon MA, Urban MK, O'Connor TZ, Barash PG. The pressure rate quotient is not an idicator of myocardial ischemia in humans. An echocardiographic study. Anesthesiology 78: 242–250, 1993
7. Flachskampf FA, Verlande M, Schneider W, Ameling W, Hanarth P. Initial experience with a multiplane transesophageal echotransducer: assessment of diagnostic potential. Eur Heart J 13: 1201–1206, 1992
8. Kolev N, Ihra G, Leitner K, Spiss CK, Zimpfer M. Improved detection of perioperative myocardial ischemia with multiplane (Hewlett Packard) transesophageal scanning: Two-dimensional biplane and transmitral Doppler echocardiography. J Cardiovasc Diag Proc (NY) (in press), 1994
9. Rafferty T. Intraoperative monitoring of ischemia and systolic cardiac function. In: Missri J, ed. Transesophageal echocardiography: clinical and intraoperative applications. Churchill Livingstone, New York, pp 181–192, 1993
10. Kolev N, Lasarova M, Lengyel M. Doppler echocardiographic determination of left ventricular output. J Cardiovasc Diag Proc (NY) 5: 146–149, 1986
11. Huemer G, Kolev N, Zimpfer M. Transesophageal echocardiographic assessment of mitral and aortic valve function during CPR. Intensive Care Med (in press) 1995
12. Kahalan MK. Transesophageal echocardiography. In: Annual Refresher Course Lectures. October 15–19, San Francisco, p 112, 1994
13. Rafferty T, LaMantia KR, Davis E, Philips D, Harris S, Carter J, Ezekowitz M, McCloskey G, Godek H, Kraker P, Jaeger D, Kopriva C, Barash P. Quality assurance for intraoperative transesophageal echocardiography monitoring: a report of 846 procedures. Anesth Analg 76: 228–232, 1993
14. Flachskampf FA, Hanrath P. Biplane and multiplane transesophageal echocardiography. In: Roelandt JRTC, Sutherland GR, Iliseto S, Linker DT, eds. Cardiac ultrasound. Curchill Livingstone, Edinburgh, pp 135–139, 1993

Chapter 4

On-line and off-line determinations of ventricular preloads and volumes

Before one can understand the clinical utility of TEE entirely it is necessary to become familiar with the applications and limitations of certain principles of cardiology. To begin with, it is important to differentiate between overall cardiac performance and myocardial contractility. Overall cardiac performance reflects the interaction of the heart, blood volume and blood vessels. These component parts together determine the extent of left ventricular fiber shortening during systole, the magnitude of ventricular wall thickness and the size of the left ventricle. Impaired overall cardiac performance can result from abnormal loading conditions (changes in blood volumes or blood pressures). These factors modify traditional indices of left ventricular function such as ejection fraction, fractional shortening, stroke volume and cardiac output. In contrast to overall cardiac performance, contractility, or inotropic state, is an intrinsic property of the myocardial muscle that leads to force generation: it can be depressed by acute ischemia, acidosis, and cardiac toxins (including medication). Overall cardiac performance reflects the interplay of preload, afterload, contractility and heart rate.

Preload - clinical relevance

Preload is classically described as the stretch applied to the left ventricle as the blood distends it at *end-diastole*.[1] If all other conditions remain unchanged, left ventricular end-diastolic volume correlates directly with stroke volume; this relationship is the basis of the Frank-Starling law of the heart (Fig. 4.1). This fundamental mechanism represents the heterometric cardiac autoregulation and refers to the intrinsic ability of the heart to adapt its performance to changes in initial muscle length, or preload. The degree of ventricular filling in diastole determines the extent to which the relaxed muscle fibers in the walls are stretched, which ultimately determines the resting length of the sarcomeres. With the ensuing contraction, the strength of muscular contraction and the extent of myocardial fibers shortening and, consequently, the stroke volume, are augmented by increases in the end-diastolic fiber length.

A variety of factors determine the end-diastolic volume of the ventricles and therefore the preload on the myocardial fibers:

a) The most important one is the status of *intravascular blood volume*. Reductions in intravascular volume[2] produced by hemorrhage or dehydration will reduce

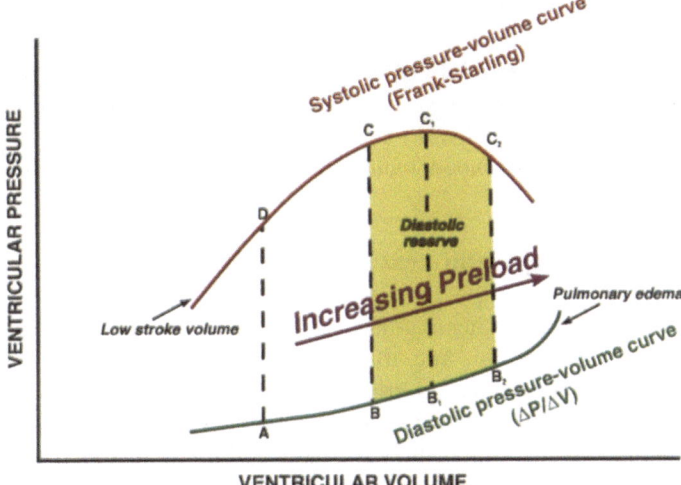

Fig. 4.1. Influence of the preload on a ventricular pressure volume relationship. An increase in ventricular preload is favorable for ventricular systolic function because of the augmentation of stroke volume through the Frank-Starling mechanism. This benefit to systolic function carries an undesirable cost in diastole, because there is an obligatory increase $\Delta P/\Delta V$. The extent of this trade-off between the potential for preload reserve to improve systolic function and the cost in the tendency to develop pulmonary edema depends on the position and the form of work diagram of the heart (i.e., pressure-volume loop; *A* mitral valve opening; *B* mitral valve closure; *C* aortic valve opening; *D* aortic valve closure) and epitomizes the important role of diastolic function

venous return and thus reduce ventricular filling, cardiac output and particularly stroke volume.

b) *Venous tone.* Increased venous tone or venoconstriction, as it occurs in states of altered sympathetic output (anxiety, marked hypotension) or with administration of sympathomimetic agents, increases the pressure gradient for venous return, thus displacing peripheral blood centrally, i.e., augmenting intrathoracic blood volume.[3] In contrast, venodilators produce extrathoracic (peripheral) pooling[3] with decrease venous return and thereby ultimately reduce preload and cardiac output.

c) *Intrathoracic pressure.* Negative intrathoracic pressure normally increases thoracic blood volume, improving cardiac filling and thereby cardiac output. Elevation of mean intrathoracic pressure, as it occurs with application of PEEP[4] or the development of pneumothorax, tend to impede total venous return to the heart, diminishing intrathoracic blood volume, and ultimately reducing cardiac output.

d) *Intrapericardial pressure.* When pericardial pressure is elevated, as occurs in pericardial effusion, there is an interference with cardiac filling, and the resulting reduction in ventricular diastolic volume (preload) decreases ventricular performance. Chronic constrictive pericarditis also impedes ventricular filling.

e) *Atrial contribution to ventricular filling.* A vigorous, appropriately timed atrial contraction augments ventricular filling and end-diastolic volumes.[1] Atrial contraction contributes relatively little to intraventricular filling in the normal heart at low heart rates. However, in pathologic states with ventricular hypertrophy (hypertension, ischemic heart disease), atrial contraction is crucial in augmenting ventricular blood volume at end-diastole, thus determining preload.

Off-line echocardiographic estimations of preload

Until the advent of TEE during anesthesia, left ventricular end-diastolic volume was difficult to measure directly, and thus preload was often derived indirectly by monitoring pulmonary artery occlusion pressure or pulmonary capillary wedge pressure (PCWP). Thus, one must assume that right ventricular end-diastolic pressure equals PCWP and that there is a close and linear relation between PCWP and right ventricular end-diastolic volume. Unfortunately, the relationship between PCWP and right ventricular end-diastolic volume is not linear and good.[5-7] Furthermore, since many patients with coronary heart disease, hypertension, ventricular hypertrophy and ventilation with PEEP have abnormal ventricular compliance, equating filling pressures with administration of volume can be misleading and may result in incorrect therapeutic decisions.[6-8]

What is the pathophysiological explanation of the fact that left ventricular end-diastolic volume cannot be substituted for PCWP in such cases? The answer has to do with ventricular **diastolic** *pressure-volume relations*, which determine *compliance*. Ventricular distensibility or compliance is the ratio of change in ventricular volume relative to change in ventricular diastolic pressure ($\Delta V/\Delta P$), while ventricular stiffness is the reciprocal or the change in pressure for a given change in volume ($\Delta P/\Delta V$).[1,9,10] The diastolic pressure-volume relation in the normal ventricle is curvilinear (Fig. 4.2). At a low ventricular end-diastolic pressure there is a relatively shallow slope, with large changes in volume being accompanied by small changes in pressure. At the upper limit of normal end-diastolic pressure, the curve becomes steeper and approximates an exponential relation, so that as the chamber becomes progressively filled, ventricular stiffness increases (i.e., compliance decreases). At this point, when the diastolic pressure-volume curve operates at its steeper part, very small changes in volume may produce large diastolic pressure changes consistent with increased stiffness. In patients with ischemic heart disease, ventricular hypertrophy, hypertension or on PEEP ventilation, diastolic pressure-volume curves ($\Delta P/\Delta V$) are steeper at lower ventricular volumes (increased stiffness); in addition, the curves are shifted upwards and to the left (Fig. 4.2). For this reason, in patients with increased ventricular stiffness, filling pressure (central venous pressure for the right ventricle and PCWP for the left ventricle) could be misleading when used for assessment of preload.

TEE echocardiography offers a practical solution for intraoperative preload assessment, because it directly images the left ventricle. Changes in left ventricular end-diastolic area are considered to reflect changes in left ventricular end-diastolic volume directly[11]; therefore TEE provides a better index of preload than pressure

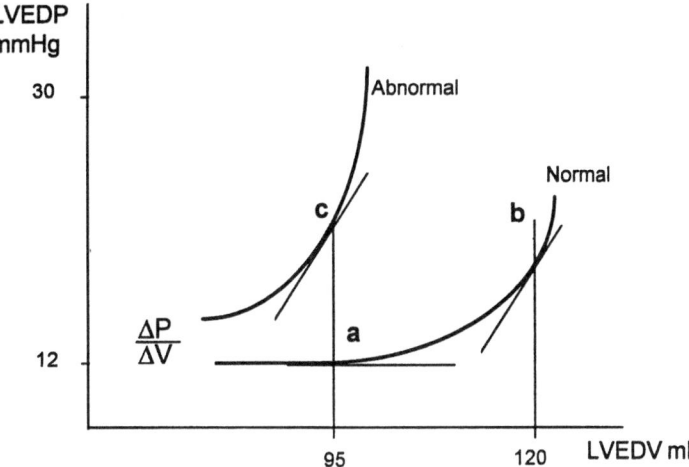

Fig. 4.2. Diagrammatic representation of left ventricular diastolic pressure-volume relationship ($\Delta P/\Delta V$) or myocardial stiffness as a tangent. At the same end-diastolic volume (95 ml) the tangent to the $\Delta P/\Delta V$ curve in a normal heart (*a*) is flattened, (decreased stiffness), while in an abnormal heart (*c*) the tangent is steepened (increased stiffness). The similarly increased stiffness in normal heart can be achieved only by augmented preload (*b*)

measurements. Thys et al.[12] and Hansen et al.[5] compared invasive hemodynamic indices with two-dimensional TEE indices during cardiac surgery; they found no correlation between PCWP and end-diastolic area or volume and concluded that PCWP did not provide reliable information about left ventricular preload. Reich et al.[13] came to a similar conclusion and demonstrated that two-dimensional TEE allows identification of mild reductions in blood volume (5–10 mm Hg decrease in systolic arterial pressure) by observing the changes in the left ventricular short-axis, with 90% sensitivity and 80% specificity.

The usefulness of preload estimation from TEE in predicting hypovolemia was compared to other routinely obtained hemodynamic parameters in 139 patients who were undergoing elective coronary artery bypass graft surgery.[14] It was found that the appearance of low cardiac volume on TEE was infrequently preceded by any acute alteration in hemodynamic parameters. Overall, only 20% of the low left ventricular volume episodes were associated with increased (greater than 10%) heart rate; with decreased systolic blood pressure, 21%; diastolic blood pressure, 25%; pulmonary artery diastolic pressure, 16%; and central venous pressure, 12%. Therefore, routine hemodynamic measurements appear to be insensitive measures of low left ventricular volume compared to TEE.

Recent studies demonstrated that two-dimensional echocardiography produces reliable estimates of left ventricular volumes if an accurate geometric model of the left ventricle is used.[15] The two basic approaches most commonly employed include:

1. *Prolate ellipse method, area-length* method—use of the volume of a single figure (prolate ellipse) to represent left ventricular volume

2. *Simpson's rule method*—the sum of multiple cross-sectional cuts to "reconstruct" the left ventricle

Prolate ellipse method, area-length approach

The single figure that has been used most extensively to represent the left ventricle is the prolate ellipsoid. This figure forms the basis for most angiographic calculation of the left ventricular volume, and its validity as a model of the left ventricle has been well documented.[15,16] The prolate ellipsoid is illustrated in Fig. 4.3 (left). This figure has two minor axes (D_1) and (D_2) and a major axis (L). It can also be sectioned through its long axis to provide orthogonal areas, or through its short axes to yield a third area. The volume of this ellipsoid can be calculated by using the following formula:

$$V = 4/3\pi \times \frac{L}{2} \times \frac{D_1}{2} \times \frac{D_2}{2} \tag{1}$$

The ellipsoid model can be applied to echocardiographic images by use of the short axis area to derive a unique echocardiographic ellipsoid area-length formula. Because the short axis area is equal to

$$\pi(D_1/2)(D_2/2) \tag{2}$$

the ellipsoid volume equation than becomes[17]

$$V = 2/3(L)(A_c) \tag{3}$$

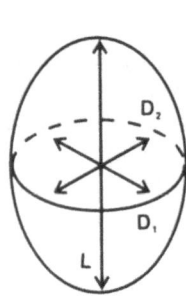
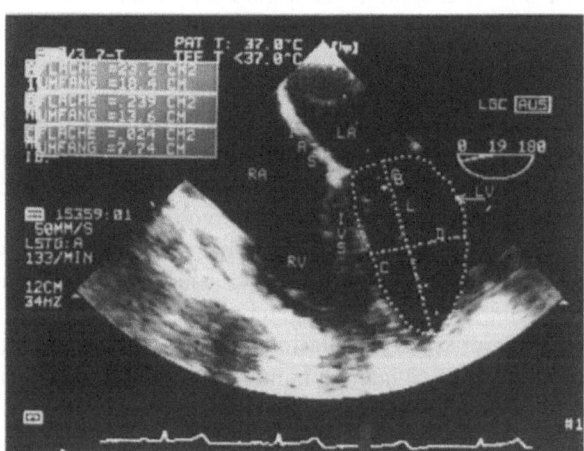

Fig. 4.3. Left: Schematic representation of the diameters of the prolate ellipse, which are used for the calculation of ventricular volumes. Right: Two-dimensional echocardiogram of the longitudinal left ventricular image, four-chamber view from midesophageal scanning. D_1 and D_2 are the minor-axis dimensions, while L is the long-axis length. *LV* left ventricle; *RV* right ventricle; *LA* left atrium; *RA* right atrium; *IVS* interventricular septum; *IAS* interatrial septum

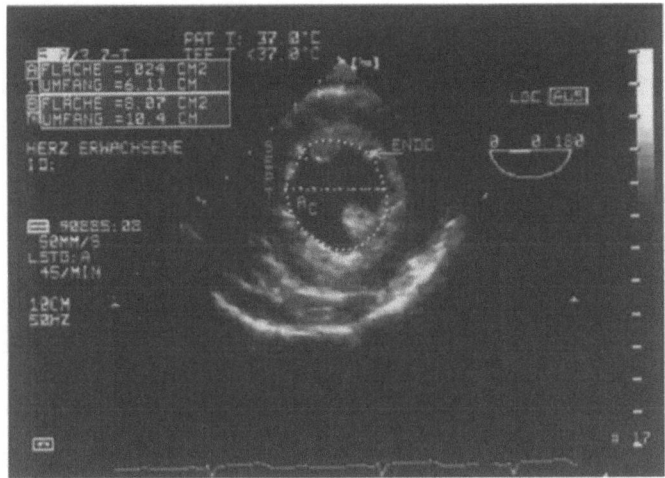

Fig. 4.4. Left ventricular short-axis view at the level of the papillary muscle representing the measurement of diameter A_c from the endocardial border

where L is estimated from a long-axis view and A_c is the area of the short-axis cross-section (Fig. 4.4).

Simpson's rule method

The principal difficulty in using the prolate ellipse model with the area-length approach is that the chamber frequently does not resemble a prolate ellipse. With any significant dyskinesis or aneurysmal dilatation, the geometric model is significantly destroyed. Even the normal ventricle does not resemble a prolate ellipse in systole. An alternative approach uses the angiographically validated method called Simpson's rule, which is integrated in the computer software of new generation echo apparatus. The superiority of this method is its reliability when ventricular geometry deviates from a prolate ellipse (for example, in dyskinesis). The mathematical basis for Simpson's rules relies on the fact that the volume of any object, regardless of shape, equals the sum of the volumes of multiple individual slices of known thickness that compose the object. Although sometimes called the "disk summation method", this method does not require that the figures be circular discs. Each of these slices can be represented by a series of ellipsoid cylinders. Thus, total left ventricular volume can be represented by the formula[15,16]:

$$V = \frac{\pi}{4} \times \frac{H}{n} \times \sum_{0}^{n} \times (D_1)(D_2) \tag{4}$$

where V = volume; H = the height of the chamber; n = number of slices; and D_1 and D_2 are the minor axis dimensions (Fig. 4.5).

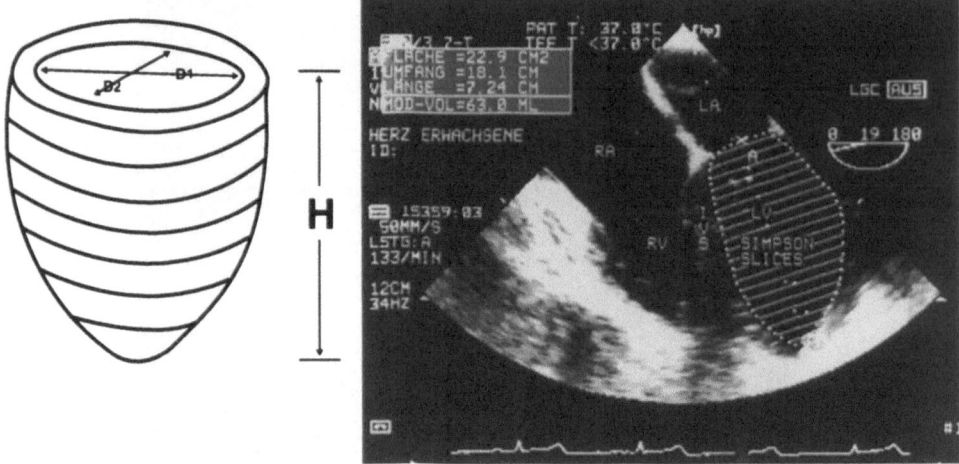

Fig. 4.5. Left: Illustration of the use of Simpson's rule to determine left ventricular volume. The chamber is represented by a series of ellipsoid cylinders. The sum of the volumes of the individual slices gives total chamber volume. Right: Two-dimensional echocardiogram of the left ventricular image, four-chamber view from midesophageal scanning. *H* height of the chamber; *D*₁ and *D*₂ are minor axis dimensions; *LV* left ventricle; *RV* right ventricle; *LA* left atrium; *RA* right atrium; *IVS* interventricular septum

The more irregularly shaped the object, the larger the number of individual slices required for accurate volume determination. Each of these slices can be represented by a series of ellipsoid cylinders (Fig. 4.5). The use of an isolated contracting canine heart preparation has shown that as the number of slices used to approximate a conical shape decreases, the more the cone resembles a cylinder. The standard error of the estimate (a predictor of accuracy of the test) fell substantially when fewer than four cross-sectional slices were used.[16] It appears therefore that at least four slices are required to get highly accurate estimates of left ventricular geometry and volume using Simpson's rule, especially if the ventricle is abnormally shaped. The Simpson's rule method is attractive as a means of calculating left ventricular volume because it avoids geometric assumptions and is usable even when ventricular shape has become markedly destroyed.

All the above-mentioned methods of volume calculation use several well-defined echocardiographic planes (longitudinal, orthogonal) from the transthoracic approach and make some permissible assumptions about three-dimensional ventricular geometry. With TEE it may be difficult to obtain a true left ventricular long-axis image, because it may not be technically possible to direct the ultrasound beam through the apex from the confines of the esophagus. The apex also lies in the far field of the sector scan and may not be well defined. Thus, a major limitation in assessing ventricular volumes using the above-described formulas by TEE is that usually only a *foreshortened* long axis (L) from a four-chamber view can be obtained in which the area that appears to be the apex is not the anatomical apex.[15,17,18] Moreover, complex models (formulas 1 and 3) requiring many planes and off-line assessment, are neither feasible nor practical for routine monitoring in the operation room. It therefore appears more logical to adopt a system using a single *short-axis* plane that *monitors changes in volume, rather than measuring volume itself.*

Previous studies have shown that changes in A_c (formula 3) rather than L more directly reflect changes in left ventricular end-diastolic volume (LVEDV). The midpapillary short-axis view (A_c) (Fig. 4.4) used in the monitoring of regional wall motion abnormalities is the best plane since at this level small changes in the position of the transducer have the smallest effect on the enclosed area of the left ventricular cavity.[18,19] Moreover, nine-tenths of the stroke volume is derived from a shortening in a ventricular short-axis. Very little contribution to the cardiac output results from shortening of the long-axis, and thus, changes in left ventricular filling cause larger changes in the short-axis dimension than in the long-axis dimension.[17] Furthermore, A_c and LVEDV have been shown to have a linear relationship over a wide range of LVEDV.[20] Consequently, changes in A_c will consistently indicate changes in LVEDV, although an individual estimate derived from A_c may be greater or less than the actual LVEDV.

Now, with advances in technology and with commercially available biplane and omniplane TEE transducers, a more accurate determination of left ventricular volumes should be possible.

A few years ago Clements and de Bruijn[19] and Cahalan et al.,[17] in agreement with ASA guidelines, recommended the use of TEE in the operating room to estimate changes in A_c as a direct indicator of changes in LVEDV, but not as a method to derive absolute LVEDV.[17]

Despite the above-mentioned limitations, anesthesia practice with echocardiography confirms that left ventricular preload is better estimated by two-dimensional TEE than by measurements of PCWP.[6-8,12,13,18-26] Normal values of left ventricular dimensions, areas and volumes using TEE are shown in Table 4.1.

Table 4.1. Normal values of left ventricle images in the TEE short-axis and four-chamber views (data from our laboratory)

TEE short-axis view		TEE long-axis (when apex is well visualized)	
DD↔cm/m²	2.5 ± 0.4	DD↔cm/m²	2.5 ± 0.5
DD↕cm/m²	2.4 ± 0.3	DD↕cm/m²	3.4 ± 0.6
DS↔cm/m²	1.6 ± 0.3	DS↔cm/m²	1.6 ± 0.4
DS↕cm/m²	1.5 ± 0.3	DS↕cm/m²	2.5 ± 0.4
EDA cm²/m²	12.9 ± 2.3		26.1 ± 3.9
ESA cm²/m²	4.7 ± 1.1		12.8 ± 3.0
EDVI ml/m²			63.5 ± 10.3
ESVI ml/m²			25.8 ± 6.7

DD diastolic diameter; *DS* systolic diameter; *EDA* end diastolic area; *ESA* end-systolic area; *EDVI* end-diastolic volume index; *ESVI* end-systolic volume index. Values are means $\pm$ 2SD.

For optimal scanning of consecutive heart beats, the patient should be in expiration. During the procedure the two-dimensional echocardiographic recordings should be digitized for slow-motion analysis. The accuracy of the results of any analysis (volume, contractility, afterload or regional wall motion pattern) can be affected significantly by tracing of the endocardial (or epicardial) outline because this procedure is prone to error in recognizing which portion of the returned ultrasound signal is actually that boundary.[27] Although the true two-dimensional endocardial edge is a discrete, vanishing small ring, echocardiographic imaging gives this border a finite degree of thickness. The gain settings of the apparatus affect this thickness, with higher gains resulting in a "thicker" boundary. Thus, a border has a leading and a trailing edge (closer to and farther from the transducer, respectively). This is especially apparent in the portions of the edge that are perpendicular to the ultrasound beam (Fig. 4.6). Tracing of the area of the endocardial cavity, for example, makes it possible to identify the boundaries of the endocardium by using any permutation of the two leading and trailing edges. However, depending on the amount of thickness given to the boundaries, a trailing edge-leading edge analysis produces different results from a leading edge-trailing edge technique. Wyatt et al.[28] studied the influence of these variations on the accuracy of linear and area measurements of echocardiograms and reported that only the leading-edge to leading-edge method resulted in acceptable correlations to direct in vitro observations. This technique involves tracing along the edge of the endocardial border closest to the transducer.[24] After outlining the end-diastolic and end-systolic contours with the track-ball, a slow motion replay is used to reevaluate the drawn contours and if the contours are not positioned correctly they can be changed.

The first step in the quantitative measurements of volumes is the selection of appropriate beats. In cases of extrasystole, only a sinus beat preceded by a sinus beat should be used for analysis in order to circumvent the problem of postextrasystolic potentiation (augmentation). End-diastole is determined as the beginning of QRS or the last frame before closure of the mitral valve.[18-21] For practical purposes it is better to use the peak of the simultaneously recorded electrocardiographic R-wave,

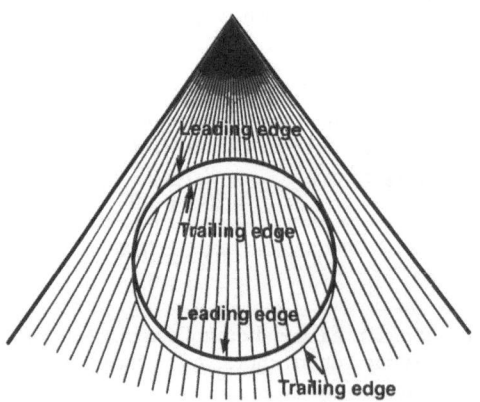

Fig. 4.6. Diagrammatic representation of the position of the leading and trailing edges of the left ventricular short-axis cross-section plane

which corresponds to the first frame with closed mitral leaflets.[18-21] As the aortic valve is not yet opened, a full contour of the ventricle is visible. End-systole is defined as the smallest left ventricular silhouette, which coincides with the last half of the electrocardiographic T-wave.[18-21] Alternatively, the beat corresponding to the closure point of the aortic valve can be chosen (if it is well visualized in the long-axis view, which is rare). Some authors use phonocardiograms to determine end-systole, but the phonocardiographic detection of end-systole has not as yet been shown to be superior to the methods mentioned above. For left ventricular volume or area determination in ventricles with dyskinesis, biplane (short-axis and long-axis views) are recommended. A minimum of 3 heart cycles in patients with sinus rhythm and 5–8 cycles in patients with atrial fibrillation should be analyzed and averaged.

In most studies comparing contrast angiographic and two-dimensionally determined left ventricular volumes, the ultrasound volumes are smaller than those calculated using invasive techniques.[15] This can be explained by the fact that radio-opaque dye used in cine angiography fills in the intertrabecular spaces, making the cardiac silhouette appear larger than it really is. This results in overestimation of true left ventricular size. On the other hand, echocardiography suffers from the inability to image the space between trabeculae. This causes incorporation of intertrabecular spaces into the endocardial borders, resulting in underestimation of true left ventricular size.[15]

Off-line measurements are valid estimates of left ventricular filling, volumes and preload, but the analysis necessary is too time-consuming to be of practical value in the operating room. In contrast, the use of an on-line automated boundary detection system can be helpful in guiding administration of fluids and inotropes.

On-line assessment of preload: acoustic quantification technique

The standard computer-based image processing procedure used for echocardiographic border detection is termed segmentation. This method automatically demarcates one region from another—for example, left ventricular blood pool cavity from myocardium—and outlines the border between these two regions.[21,32-36] In general, this method compares information received from each pictures element (pixel) to an established "threshold value."[21] The currently available automated boundary detection (ABD) system uses a computer algorithm that analyzes unprocessed radiofrequency or acoustic signals in real time at each pixel along all lines. Then acoustic information is converted into a power signal, which is compared with a threshold value in order to discriminate blood from tissue. Boundary points are finally assigned and connected in order to form a continuous border, which is superimposed on the conventional two-dimensional image. The ABD Hewlett Packard (Acoustic Quantification, Andover, MA) *Sonos* 1500 and *Sonos* 2500 determine transition points between blood and myocardium, marking them with a highlighted border indicator or in a solid red color—blood format.

Conventional two-dimensional echocardiographic images are acquired carefully to optimize the delineation of the endocardial borders, and the automated boundary detection system is activated. When the border alignment is not satisfactory, the operator must readjust transmit control, time gain control (TGC) and lateral gain control (LGC). In general, excess gain results in an underestimation of cavity area and insufficient gain results in poor tracking.[21,37,38]

Next, a region of interest (ROI) is defined and outlined with a trackball; the ROI includes all portions of the systolic and diastolic frames of the border surrounding the structure of interest (i.e., just outside the left ventricular epicardial border). Thus, ROI should include all of the targeted blood area, but should exclude the blood area that one does not want to be measured (Fig. 4.7). Some use blood format when the ROI must be defined, but actually both types of border detection are equal in their capabilities in border detection.

ABD sums the cross-sectional area of blood in each video frame and displays this information as continuously updated points of the systolic and diastolic cross-sectional areas and derived variables, such as the ejection fraction area [(end-diastolic area—end-systolic area)/end-diastolic area]. Additionally, the first derivative of the area changes with respect to time in cm^2/sec (dA/dt) can be obtained by means of a special resistance-capacitance circuit (Fig. 4.7). Positive peak of dA/dt occurs and represents the peak filling rate of the left ventricle.[21] Moreover, time from peak of QRS to the peak of the first derivative of volume change, i.e., t-peak filling rate,[21] which has a physiological significance similar to t-peak dP/dt, is displayed on the screen.

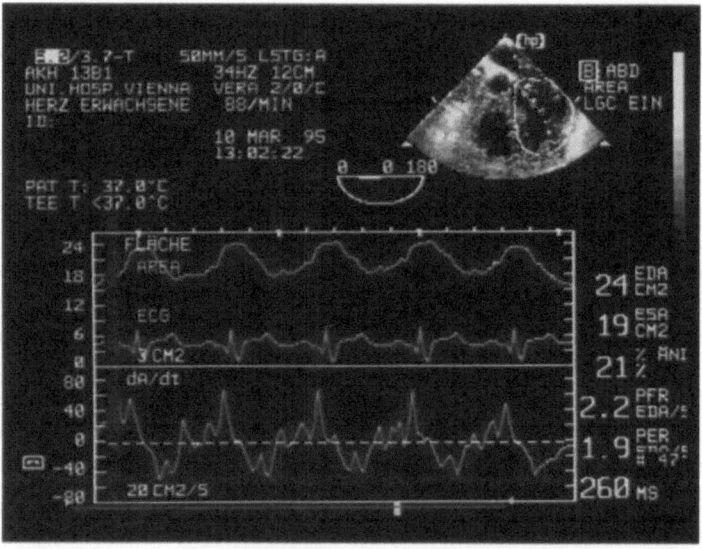

Fig. 4.7. A split-screen image showing left ventricular midesophageal four-chamber long-axis view with activated automatic boundary detection system and outlined region of interest. The calculations are given in two waves, namely, the area of the left ventricle and its first derivative, dA/dt, as well as in numerical values of end-diastolic area (*EDA*), end-systolic area (*ESA*), percent change of area, i.e., ejection fraction area (*ANI*), peak filling rate (*PFR*) positive peak dA/dt, peak ejection rate (*PER*) negative peak dA/dt, and time to peak positive dA/dt. ECG is reference curve

In 80% of cases, ABD estimates end-diastolic and end-systolic borders within the expected limits, when verified by an expert.[21,32] In the other 20% of cases, difficulties with ABD tracing or cavity area estimation are confirmed also by viewing the real-time images. Thus, ABD performance is critically dependent on the quality of TEE images, which, in turn, depend on the skill of the operator in producing high-resolution TEE images.[33-35] Anesthesiologists currently using the ABD system need to be aware of this limitation set by image quality and gain setting inherent in the early phase of application.

On-line ABD has some other limitations. Small areas of left ventricular myocardium in the septum and lateral wall frequently are identified as blood and not tissue because most of the myocytes within these walls are oriented parallel to the ultrasound beam, and therefore reflect less ultrasound than do structures oriented perpendicular to the beam.[32] Furthermore, there are important differences in the method of quantification used by the ABD system compared with that of conventional manual measurements. In the former, papillary muscles are excluded from the cavity area because ABD correctly recognizes them as tissue and not blood.[21,33] Nevertheless, using off-line estimation, some authors included papillary muscles,[33,39] excluded them,[40] or did not specify them at all.[41]

Despite these insignificant limitations ABD system provides a reliable, real-time estimation of left ventricular end-diastolic and end-systolic area and volume,[42] displaying them as a waveform that gives instantaneous beat-by-beat information about left ventricular preload and ejection fraction area, in the operating room. The latter data are invaluable (much more than invasive data) for swift therapeutic decision at time of operation, when the patient develops suddenly hypotension (Table 4.2).

Table 4.2. Diagnosis of the causes for *hypotension* with ABD system

LVEDA	EFA	Diagnosis
↓	↑	hypovolemia
↑	↓	myocardial depression or ischemia
↔	↑	low systemic resistance

LVEDA left ventricular end-diastolic area; *EFA* ejection fraction area.

Moreover, on-line evaluation of left ventricular volumes and areas has the clear advantage over off-line, of avoiding loss of information due to video recording.[21,34] This technology should enhance the widespread acceptance of TEE as a monitoring technique.[23,31] However, practical clinical utility of automated endocardial outlining for continuous monitoring remains to be determined.

References

1. Braunwald E, Sonnenblick EH, Ross J Jr. Mechanisms of cardiac contraction and relaxation. In: Braunwald E, ed. Heart Disease, 4th ed.WB Saunders, Philadelphia, pp 379–391, 1992

2. Guyton AC. Textbook of medical physiology. 8th ed, WB Saunders, Philadelphia, p 227, 1991

3. Sheferd JT, Vanhoutte PM. Veins and their control. WB Saunders, Philadelphia, p 269, 1987

4. Huemer G, Kolev N, Kurz A, Zimpfer M. Influence of positive end-expiratory pressure on right and left ventricular performance assessed by Doppler two-dimensional echocardiography. Chest 106: 67–73, 1994

5. Hansen RM, Viquerat CE, Matthay MA, Wiener-Kronish JP, DeMarko T, Bahtta S, Marks JD, Botwinick EH, Chatterjee K. Poor correlation between pulmonary arterial wedge pressure and left ventricular end-diastolic volume after coronary artery bypass graft surgery. Anesthesiology 64: 764–770, 1986

6. Cheatham ML, Chang MC, Eddy VA, Safcsak K, Nelson LD. Right ventricular end-diastolic volume index and pulmonary artery occlusion pressure vs cardiac index in patients on positive end-expiratory pressure (Abstr). Crit Care Med 22: A98, 1994

7. Godje O, Schwab R, Zimmermann G, Blumel G, Reihart B, Pfeiffer U. Discrepancy between left ventricular enddiastolic pressure and pulmonary wedge pressure during mechanical ventilation (Abstr). Crit Care Med 22: A100, 1994

8. Van Aken H, Vandermeersch E. Reliability of PCWP as an index for left ventricular preload. Br J Anesth 60 [Suppl 1]: 85S–89S, 1988

9. Kolev N, Zimpfer M. Impact of myocardial ischemia on diastolic function: Clinical relevance and recent Doppler echocardiographic insights. Eur J Anaesth 11 (in press), 1994

10. Kolev N, Uzunov G, Vlaskov V. Hemodynamic and pharmacologic influences on the left ventricular echo dimension-pressure loops in dogs. J Cardiography (Tokyo) 14: 537–542, 1984

11. De Bruijn NP, Clements FM. Transesophageal echocardiography. Martinus Nijhoff, Boston, pp 94–97, 1987

12. Thys DM, Hillel Z, Goldman ME, Mindich BP, Kaplan JA. A comparison of hemodynamic indices derived by invasive monitoring and two-dimensional echocardiography. Anesthesiology 67: 630–634, 1987

13. Reich DL, Konstandt SN, Abrams HP, Buseck J. Intraoperative transesophageal echocardiography for detection of cardiac preload changes induced by transfusion and phlebotomy in pediatric patients. Anesthesiology 79: 10–15, 1993

14. Leung JM, Chan FW, Mangano DT. Transesophageal echocardiography: Prediction of intraoperative hypovolemia (Abstr). Anesth Analg 70: S263, 1990

15. Erbel R. Principles of global left ventricular function analysis. In: Roelandt JRTC, Sutherland GR, Iliceto S, Linker DT, eds. Cardiac ultrasound. Churchill Livinstone, Edinburgh, London, pp 219–231, 1993

16. Borow K. Integrated approach to the noninvasive assessment of left ventricular systolic and diastolic performance. In: St John Sutton M, Oldershaw PJ, eds. Textbook of adult and pediatric echocardiography and Doppler. Blackwell, Boston, pp 97–115, 1989

17. Cahalan MK, Lurz FC, Schiller NB. Transesophageal two-dimensional echocardiographic evaluation of anaesthetic effects on left ventricular function. Br J Anaesth 60: 99S–106S, 1988

18. van Daele MERM, Roelamdt JRTC. Intraoperative monitoring. In: Sutherland GR, Roelandt JRTC, Fraser A, Anderson RH, eds. Transesophageal echocardiography in clinical practice. Gower London, pp 12.7–12.16, 1991

19. Clements FM, de Bruijn NP. Perioperative evaluation of regional wall motion by transesophageal two-dimensional echocardiography. Anesth Analg 66: 249–261, 1987

20. Takahashi M, Sasayama S, Kavai C, Kotoura H. Contractile performance of the hypertrophied ventricle in patients with systemic hypertension. Circulation 62: 116–126, 1980

21. Kolev N, Huemer G, Steiner W, Leitner K. On-line assessment of left ventricular volumes and ejection fraction by automatic boundary detection and backscatter ultrasound image. J Cardiovasc Diag Proc (NY) 11: 141–145, 1993

22. Kikura M, Shanewise JS, Levy JH. Intraoperative assessment of myocardial function. Curr Opin Anesth 7: 42–52, 1994

23. Fontes ML, Leung J, Mangano DT, SPI Research Group. Should transesophageal echocardiography monitoring be used routinely in the cardiac intensive care unit? (Abstr)Anesthesiology 79: A288, 1993

24. Clements FM, Harpole DH, Quill T, Jones RH, McCann RL. Estimation of left ventricular volumes and ejection fraction by two-dimensional echocardiography: Comparison of short axis imaging and simultaneous radionuclide angiography. Br J Anaesth 64: 331–336, 1990

25. Greim C, Roewer N, Laux G, Schulte J. Perioperative assessment of myocardial contractility by transesophageal echocardiography (Abstr). Anesthesiology 79: A547, 1993

26. Cheung AT, Savino JS, Weiss SJ. Echocardiographic and hemodynamic determinations of left ventricular preload during graded hypovolemia (Abstr). Anesthesiology 79: A83, 1993

27. Stanley TE. Quantitative echocardiography. In: de Bruijn NP, Clements FM, eds. Intraoperative use of echocardiography. Lippincott, Philadelphia, pp 59–73, 1991

28. Wyatt HL, Haensechen RV, Meerbaum S. Assessment of quantitative methods for two-dimensional echocardiography. Am J Cardiol 52: 396–401, 1983

29. Cahalan MK, Ionescu P, Melton HE, Adler S, Kee LL, Schiller NB. Automated analysis of intraoperative transesophageal echocardiograms. Anesthesiology 78: 477–485, 1993

30. Perez JE, Waggoner AD, Barzilai B, Melton HJ, Miller JG, Sobel BE. On-line assessment of ventricular function by automatic boundary detection and ultrasonic bacckscatter imaging. J Am Coll Cardiol 19: 313–320, 1992

31. Duft S, Greim C, Roewr N, Laux G, Schulte J. Echocardiographic assessment of fractional area change by halothane: automatic vs manual quantification (Abstr). Anesth Analg 78: S100, 1994

32. Melton HJ, Collins SM, Skorton DJ. Automatic real-time endocardial edge detection in two-dimensional echocardiography. Ultrasound Imaging 5: 300–307, 1993

33. Cahalan MK, Weiskopf RB, Egger II EI, Yasuda N, Ionescu P, Rampil IJ, Lockhart SH, Freire B, Peterson NA. Hemodynamic effect of desflurane/nitrous oxide anesthesia in volunteers. Anesth Analg 73: 157–164, 1991

34. Geiser EA, Oliver LH, Gardin JM, Kreber RE, Parisi AF, Reichek N, Werner JA, Weyman AE. Clinical validation of an edge detection algorithm for two-dimensional echocardiographic short axis images. J Am Soc Echocardiogr 1: 410–421, 1988

35. Geiser EA, Conetti DA, Limacher MC, Stockton VO, Oliver LH, Jones B. A second generation computer assisted edge detection algorithm for short axis two-dimensional echocardiography. J Am Soc Echocardiogr 3: 79–90, 1990

36. Markus RH, Bednarz J, Coulden R, Shroff S, Lipton M, Lang RM. Ultrasonic backsscatter system for automated on-line endocardial boundary detection: evaluation by ultrafast computed tomography. J Am Coll Cardiol 22: 839–847, 1993

37. Lindower PD, Rath L, Perslar J, Burns TL, Rezai K, Vandenberg BF. Quantification of left ventricular function with an automated border detection system and comparison with radionuclide ventriculography. Am J Cardiol 73: 195–199, 1994

38. Foster E, Cahalan MK. The search for intelligent quantitation in echocardiography: "eyball", "trackball" and beyond. J Am Coll Cardiol 22: 848–850, 1993

39. Smith JS, Roizen MF, Cahalan MK, Benefiel DJ, Beaupe PN, Sohn YJ, Schiller NB, Stoney RJ, Ehrenfeld WK. Does anesthetic technique make a difference? Augmentation of systolic blood pressure during carotid endarterectomy: Effect of phenyephrine versus light anesthesia and of isoflurane versus halothane on the incidence of myocardial ischemia. Anesthesiology 69: 846–853, 1988

40. Triulzi M, Weyman A. Normal cross-sectional measurements in adults. In: Echocardiography, Weyman A, ed. Lea & Febiger, Philadelphia, pp 497–499, 1982

41. Himelman RB, Cassidy MM, Landzberg JS, Schiller NB. Reproducibility of quantitative echocardiography. Am Heart J 115: 425–431, 1988

42. Gorcsan J, Morita S, Mandarino WA, Deneault LG, Kawai A, Kormos RL, Griffith BP, Pinsky MR. Two-dimensional echocardiographic automated border detection accurately reflects changes in left ventricular volume. J Am Soc Echocardiogr 6: 482–489, 1993

Chapter 5

Assessment of afterload

Clinical relevance

Afterload can be thought of as the *tension* acting on the fibers *in the ventricular wall during ejection* or as the impedance to ejection.[1] Although it is influenced importantly by the arterial pressure, it is not synonymous with peripheral arterial pressure, peripheral vascular tone, or systemic vascular resistance. Afterload is best defined as left ventricular wall stress during ejection according to La Place's law:[2]

$$\text{Wall stress} = \text{PR}/\text{2h}, \tag{1}$$

where P is the intracavitary pressure, R is the radius of curvature, and h is the wall thickness. Thus, wall stress is directly related to chamber dimension, and inversely related to wall thickness. While arterial pressure is related to the product of cardiac output and systemic vascular resistance, afterload (wall stress) is a function of ventricular size and arterial pressure. Fig. 5.1. illustrates the great difference between wall stress, i.e., afterload, and systolic ventricular pressure.

In anesthesia practice systemic vascular resistance (SVR) has been used to assess afterload,[3] relating to the formula:

$$\text{SVR} = (\text{MAP} - \text{CVP})/\text{CO}, \tag{2}$$

where MAP = mean arterial pressure, CVP = central venous pressure and CO = cardiac output. Because each parameter of the equation (2) has its own source of error, systemic vascular resistance does not directly reflect a change in left ventricular afterload.[4] Systemic vascular resistance is a derived hemodynamic parameter that is not routinely indexed. In comparison to systemic vascular resistance, left ventricular end-systolic stress is a more preferable index of afterload, reflecting the combined effects of intrinsic cardiac properties and peripheral loading conditions.

Although many anesthesiologists may be unfamiliar with methods of measuring wall stress using echocardiography, it is important for us to understand the basic concept of wall stress calculation because of its advantage in clinical applications. The simplest calculation of wall stress in a thin-walled spherical model based on the La Place relation is given in formula (1). For a spherical model, meridional wall stress and circumferential wall stress are equal; however, for an ellipsoid model (like the left ventricular chamber), the circumferential stress generally exceeds the meridional stress.[5]

During the ejection phase of the cardiac cycle, the left ventricular dimension decrease while pressure and wall thickness increase (Fig. 5.2). Normally, left

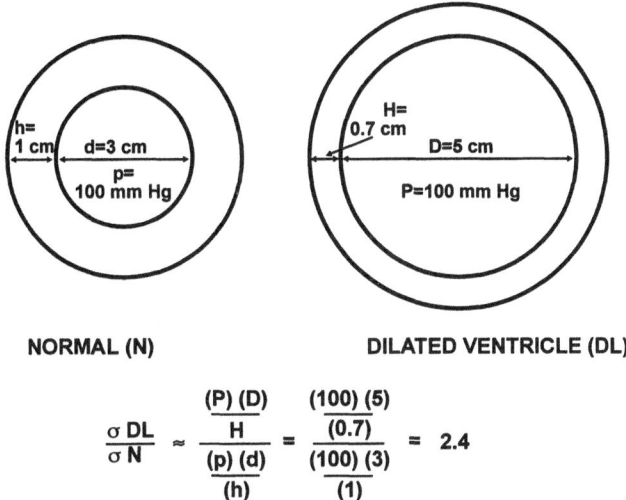

Fig. 5.1. Comparison of calculated wall stress values for a normal left ventricle (N) versus a dilated ventricle (DL). Despite the same intracavitary pressure (i.e., p = 100 mm Hg) the dimensions (d, D) and wall thickness (h, H) are quite different. This results in much higher wall stress for the dilated ventricle

ventricular wall stress reaches its peak within the first one third of the ejection phase and then declines throughout the remainder of systole (Fig. 5.2). This occurs despite rising pressures throughout most of the ejection period and emphasizes the importance of the decline in left ventricular size and the increase in wall thickness as determinants of instantaneous systolic wall stress. In the normal ventricle left ventricular end-systolic wall stress is generally less than 50% of the peak value.

Meridional wall stress measures the force acting on left ventricular fibers along the chamber's *longitudinal* axis (Fig. 5.3) and requires only measurements of the short axis. However, *circumferential* wall stress measures the forces acting on the left ventricle wall along its *minor* axis (Fig. 5.3) and thus requires measurements of the left ventricular long axis.[6,7] If a clinical echocardiographic calculation of *circumferential* wall stress is to be undertaken, the left ventricular long-axis is assumed to be twice a left ventricular short-axis cross-section. These assumptions are likely to introduce error, however, when morphological changes occur as a result of chronic left ventricular hypertrophy and/or dilatation, or when the ratio of the long axis to the short axis changes under variable conditions.

In contrast to these limitations of the *circumferential* wall stress, **meridional** wall stress does not requires a measurement of left ventricular long axis and can be estimated using the angiographically validated and clinically echocardiographically proven formula:[4,7,8]

$$\textit{Meridional}\textbf{ wall stress }(\sigma) = \frac{1.35 \times \mathbf{P} \times \mathbf{ESD}}{4h(1 + h/ESD)} \qquad (3)$$

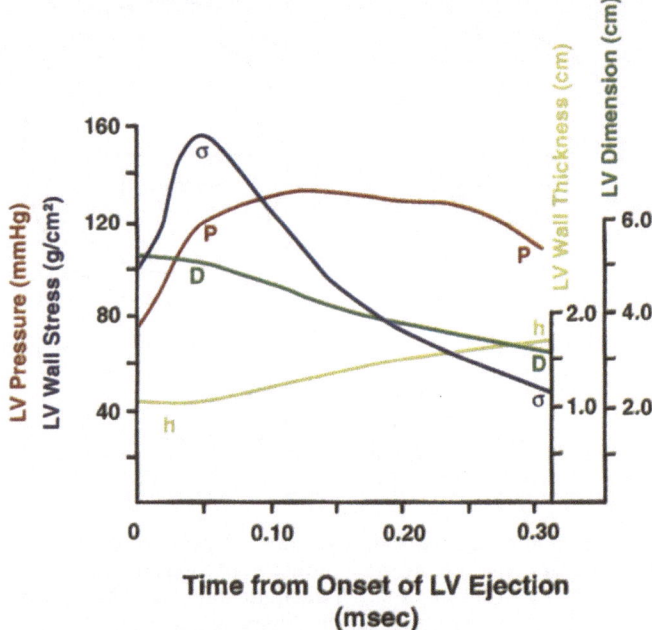

Fig. 5.2. Left ventricular wall stress (σ) i.e., afterload calculated over the course of ejection from simultaneously measurements of left ventricular pressure (P), dimension (D), and wall thickness (h) in a normal subject. Systolic wall stress peaks soon after onset of ejection and then declines throughout the remainder of systole

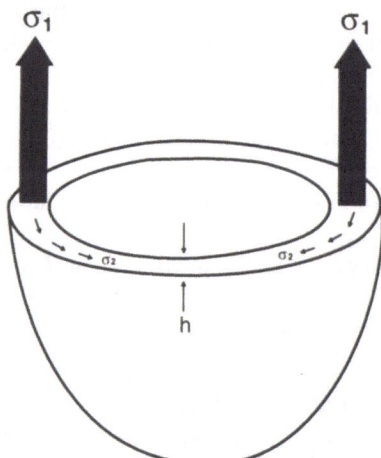

Fig. 5.3. Stylized representation of the left ventricular short-axis cross-section. Meridional wall stress, σ_1, measures the force acting along the chamber's longitudinal axis and requires only estimations of the short-axis, whereas circumferential wall stress, σ_2, measures the forces acting along the chamber's minor axis and requires estimation of long axis. h wall thickness

where P = left ventricular end-systolic pressure, ESD = left ventricular short-axis cross-section dimension at end-systole and h = left ventricular wall thickness at end-systole. Therefore, meridional wall stress has been used by several investigators, including anesthesiologists who attempted to examine rapid changes in wall stress during dynamic left ventricular loading conditions.[7-12]

Wall stress is directly related to the shape of the ventricle, which changes during the cardiac cycle and also in pathological state (heart failure, acute ischemia, cardiomyopathies etc.). At the end of systole, circumferential stress exceeds meridional stress, with their normal ratio being 2.6[13] In the above mentioned pathological states, however, as the ventricle becomes more spherical, meridional stress increases more than the circumferential stress, and their ratio decreases toward a value of 1. It has been reported to be 1.7 in a group with congestive cardiomyopathy.[13]

The use of wall stress as a measure of myocardial function is based on the principle that, for equilibrium to exist at any point of the cardiac cycle, the forces acting within the ventricular wall must exactly balance the force acting on the wall. When the ventricular function is normal an elevation in afterload reduces ventricular systolic emptying, thus increasing the end-diastolic volume, i.e., preload. The augmented preload enhances myocardial performance and tends to counteract the effect of increased afterload (Fig. 5.4). In contrast, in a failing, dilated ventricle, myocardial performance cannot be enhanced by increases in preload, so this compensatory mechanism is lost. In such cases afterload becomes an increasingly important determinant of cardiac performance,[1] because an increase in afterload may further reduce cardiac output; on the other hand, pharmacological reduction of afterload may be beneficial in elevating stroke volume.

The integral of left ventricular systolic wall stress over the ejection period, along with the heart rate and contractile state, constitute the primary determinants of myocardial oxygen consumption.[1,6] Afterload is a major determinant of myocardial oxygen consumption.[14] Smith et al.[14] reported that an intraoperative increase in systolic wall stress was related to a higher incidence of myocardial ischemia. They concluded that if afterload is evaluated by arterial pressure alone, myocardial ischemia may be overlooked.

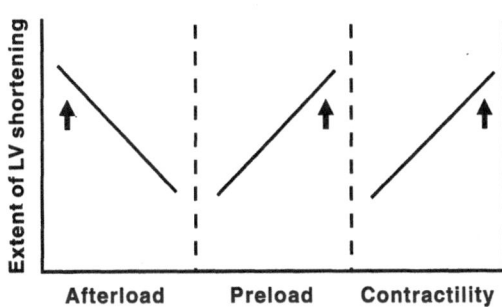

Fig. 5.4. As shown by arrows, decreased afterload, increased preload and augmented contractility can result in identical overall left ventricular performance (i.e., extent of left ventricular shortening)

Echocardiographic estimation of afterload

In anesthesia settings, afterload, according to the La Place's law (formula 3), can be determined noninvasively using echocardiography and arterial blood pressure:[11,14-16]

$$\sigma = 1.35 \times P \times ESD/4h(1 + h/ESD),$$

where σ = left ventricular meridional wall stress (g/cm^2), P = left ventricular end-systolic pressure, replaced by end-systolic arterial pressure in g/cm^2 (mm Hg $\times$ 1.35 = g/cm^2), HESD = left ventricular end-systolic dimension in short-axis cross-section (cm) and h = left ventricular end-systolic wall thickness (cm).

In cardiac mechanics it is well known that the external arterial carotid pulse contour (like the aortic one, Fig. 6.8) closely parallels the time course and magnitude of the left ventricular pressure curve during left ventricular ejection in the absence of aortic outflow tract pathology (Fig. 5.5). Accordingly, by the method of Borow and Neumann[17,18] end-systolic pressure can be measured noninvasively using calibrated carotid pulse tracings. Calibration of the carotid pulse tracing is performed by simultaneously obtaining upper arm cuff pressure and assigning systolic blood pressure to the peak and diastolic pressure to the nadir of the tracing (Fig. 5.6). Linear interpolation to the level of the dicrotic notch is then performed to estimate end-systolic pressure.

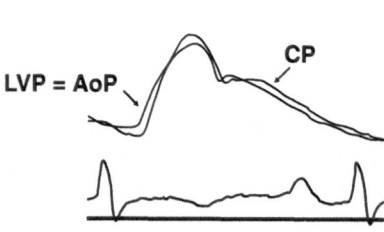

Fig. 5.5. Comparison of directly measured central aortic pressure (which, during ejection time is equal to left ventricular pressure) and external carotid pulse tracing. Note the similarity of these two curves, which permits calibrated external carotid pulse tracing to be substituted for left ventricular pressure during the ejection period. *AoP* central aortic pressure; *LVP* left ventricular pressure; *CP* external carotid pulse tracing

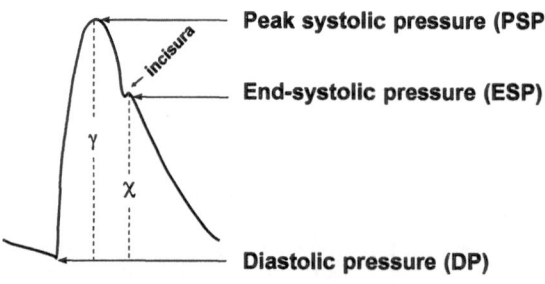

Fig. 5.6. Method for blood pressure calibration of the carotid pulse tracing. See text for explanation

Attempts to simplify data acquisition by substituting peak systolic pressure for end-systolic pressure are complicated by numerous theoretical as well as physiological problems. For example, if one uses a combination of *peak* systolic blood pressure and *end*-systolic left ventricular dimension and wall thickness in calculating wall stress, variables from *two different times* in the cardiac cycle are incorporated. The result is an apparent wall stress value approximately twofold higher than the actual value for meridional wall stress (normal values of left ventricular meridional wall stress using end-systolic pressure are $44 \pm 12 \, \text{g/cm}^2$).

Average end-systolic wall thickness (h) is derived from a two-dimensional echocardiographic short-axis view at the level of the papillary muscles. From this image the planimetered end-systolic epicardial and endocardial areas (Fig. 5.7) are obtained using the formula:[15]

$$h = \frac{\sqrt{\text{area epicardium}}}{\pi} - \frac{\sqrt{\text{area endocardium}}}{\pi}$$

Average end-systolic endocardial diameter (D) is derived from the formula:

$$D = 2 \times \frac{\sqrt{\text{area endocardim}}}{\pi}$$

Calculating wall stress requires the assumption that the radius of curvature of the left vermicular cross-section (A_c) is equal along the whole perimeter. This is clearly invalid in patients with regional systolic wall motion abnormalities. Regional wall

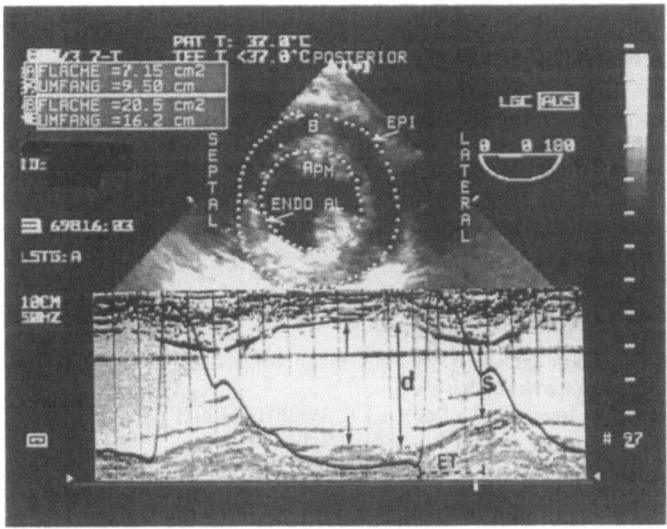

Fig. 5.7. Split-screen transesophageal two-dimensional echocardiogram of the left ventricular short-axis at the level of the papillary muscle at end-systole (top) and simultaneously recorded carotid pulse tracing using M-mode (bottom) obtained from a representative patient for calculating afterload (Hewlett Packard, Sonos 2500). *ENDO* endocard; *EPI* epicard, *d* end-diastolic diameter; *ET* ejection time; *s* end-systolic diameter

stress in this case can be calculated, based on a modified formula developed by Janz:[19,20]

$$\sigma = \frac{P \times R \times [2 - \times \sin \phi]}{2h \times \sin \phi [R + (h/2)]}$$

where P is end-systolic arterial pressure, R is the end-systolic radius of A_c, h is end-systolic wall thickness, and ϕ is the angle between R and the imaginary end-systolic radius of A_c corresponding to the dysfunctional area (i.e., the axis of asymmetry).

Ideally, calculation of wall stress is made by using simultaneous two-dimensional left ventricular short-axis images, carotid pulse tracings and the electrocardiogram. This can be accomplished by means of the split-screen format of two-dimensional and M-mode echocardiogram on which there are possibilities for simultaneous records of carotid pulse tracing, electrocardiogram as well as phonocardiogram (5.7.). In such cases the image of left ventricular dimension can be stopped exactly at the time of end-systole, i.e., at the time of the incisura of the carotid pulse tracing, taking into account the pulse transmission time (time from aortic component of the second heart sound to the incisura).

This sophisticated calculation of wall stress can be made off-line with computer-assisted video systems in research settings. With future technological advances, we believe that automated on-line assessment of wall stress will become possible. Thus, TEE should allow much better evaluation of left ventricular function during anesthesia than do other techniques.

References

1. Braunwald E, Sonnenblick EH, Ross J Jr. Mechanisms of cardiac contraction and relaxation. In: Braunwald E, ed, Heart disease. 4th ed. WB Saunders, Philadelphia, pp 351–418, 1992
2. Goertz AW, Lindner KH, Seefeld C, Schirmer U, Beyer M, Georgieff M. Effect of phenylephrine bolus administration on global left ventricular function in patients with coronary artery disease and patients with valvular aortic stenosis. Anesthesiology 78: 834–841, 1993
3. Kaplan JA. Cardiac Anesthesia. 3rd ed. Grune and Stratton, New York, London, pp 1178, 1991
4. Kikura M, Shanewise JS, Levy JH. Intraoperative assessment of myocardial function. Curr Opin Anesth 4: 42–52, 1993
5. Grossman W, Jones D, McLaurin LP. Wall stress and patterns of hypertrophy in the human left ventricle. J Clin Invest 56: 56–64, 1975
6. Lang LM, Briller RA, Neumann A, Borow KM. Assessment of afterload. In: Kreber RE, ed, Echocardiography in coronary artery disease. Future, Mount Kiosk, pp 224–225, 1988
7. Quinones MA, Mokotoff DM, Nouri S, Winters WL, Miller RR. Noninvasive quantification of left ventricular wall stress. Validation of the method and application to assessment of chronic pressure overload. Am J Cardiol 45: 782–790, 1980
8. Huemer G, Kolev N, Kurz A, Zimpfer M. Influence of positive end-expiratory pressure on right and left ventricular performance assessed by Doppler two-dimensional echocardiography. Chest 106: 67–73, 1994

9. Colan SD, Borow KM, Neumann A. Effects of loading conditions and contractile state (methoxamine and dobutamine) on left ventricular early diastolic function in normal subjects. Am J Cardiol 55: 790–796, 1985

10. Reichek N, Wilson J, St J Sutton M, Plappert TA, Goldberg S, Hirshfeld JW. Noninvasive determination of left ventricular end-systolic stress: validation of the method and initial application. Circulation 65: 99–108, 1982

11. Kikura M, Ikeda T, Kazman T, Ikeda K. Effect of prostaglandin E_1 on myocardial contractility in dogs anesthetized with halothane: Load-independent and noninvasive assessment using transesophageal echocardiography. J Cardiothorac Vasc Anesth 6: 586–592, 1992

12. Kikura M, Ikeda K. Comparison of effects of sevoflurane-nitrous oxide and enflurane-nitrous oxide on myocardial contractility in humans: load-independent and noninvasive assessment with transesophageal echocardiography. Anesthesiology 79: 235–243, 1993

13. Douglas PS. Comparison of echocardiographic methods for measurement of left ventricular shortening and wall stress. J Am Coll Cardiol 9: 945–949, 1987

14. Smith JS, Benefiel DJ, Beaupre PN, Sohn YJ, Lurz FW, Bird B, Bouchard A, Schiller NB, Cahalan MC, Roizen MF. Effects of phenylephrine on myocardial performance during carotid endarterectomy (Abstr). Anesthesiology 61: A56, 1984

15. O'Kelly BF, Tubau JF, Knight AA, London MJ, Verrier ED, Mangano DT. Measurement of left ventricular contractility using transesophageal echocardiography in patients undergoing coronary artery bypass grafting. Am Heart J 122: 1041–1048, 1991

16. Cunningham AJ, Turner J, Grosso L, Rosenbaum S, Rafferty T. Transesophageal assessment of hemodynamic function during laparoscopic cholecystectomy (Abstr). Anesth Analg 76: S64, 1993

17. Colan SD, Borow KM, Neumann A. The left ventricular end-systolic wall stress- velocity of the fiber shortening relation: A load independent index of myocardial contractility. J Am Coll Cardiol 4: 715–719, 1984

18. Colan SD, Borow KM, Neumann A. Use of the calibrated pulse tracing for calculation of left ventricular pressure and wall stress throughout ejection. Am Heart J 109: 1306–1310, 1985

19. Janz RF. Estimation of local myocardial stress. Am J Physiol 242: H875, 1982

20. Kolev N, Huemer G, Ihra G, Spiss CS, Zimpfer M. Assessment of afterload in case of regional systolic abnormalities. Int J Anaesth (in press), 1995

Chapter 6

Contractility

Contractility indices revisited

When preload and afterload are kept constant, stroke volume is dependent on contractility, or the *inotropic state* of the myocardium.[1] The inotropic state of the myocardium is an intrinsic property that reflects the strength of the muscle fiber, which in turn is influenced by the neurohormonal (especially cardiac sympathetic nerves) and metabolic (pH, Ca^{++}, etc.) milieu. Traditionally, a change in contractility in the intact heart can be defined as an alteration in overall cardiac performance that occurs independently of alterations in preload, afterload or heart rate. Because of the latter confounding variables, it has been difficult to assess left ventricular contractility in humans and particularly in the acute change of settings in surgery.[2-3]

Recently, several indices of left ventricular performance that relate to physiological events measured at end-systole have been shown to be independent of ventricular loading conditions, and thus are useful as clinical measures of contractility in anesthesia settings.[2-7] The relationship between two-dimensional echo left ventricular area and end-systolic wall stress (derived from arterial blood pressure and echo dimension) may be promising for the future.[2]

Traditional parameters of left ventricular systolic performance that can be obtained by means of TEE are:

I. *Indices for overall cardiac performance*
   A. Ejection phase indices
      1. Cardiac output or work output
      2. Ejection fraction or percent area change
      3. Mean velocity of circumferential fiber shortening (Vcf)
   B. Isovolumic phase indices
      1. Peak positive dP/dt
      2. Isovolumic contraction time (IVCT)[8]
II. *Frank-Starling principle and end-systolic indices (integrated approach)*
      1. Relationship of end-systolic volume to peak systolic pressure[4]
      2. Relationship of end-systolic area to peak systolic pressure[3]
      3. Relationship of end-systolic area to end-systolic wall stress[2]
      4. Relationship of Vcf to wall stress (σ)[6]

The ejection phase indices measure overall left ventricular performance using data collected during ventricular ejection. In general, they are dependent on preload, afterload, heart rate and contractility. As such, they are unable to distinguish abnormalities in the contractile state from compensatory or detrimental alterations in loading conditions.[1]

The isovolumic phase indices of left ventricular performance that can be obtained by means of echocardiography practically are first derivatives of the left ventricular pressure, dP/dt. Additionally, by means of Doppler echocardiography can be obtained isovolumic contraction time. The major limitation of these indices is their sensitivity to left ventricular preload as well as low aortic pressures, especially in patients with heart failure.[1]

The Frank-Starling low of the heart is the classic method used to assess left ventricular systolic performance. Recently a slightly different methods have been introduced, namely using end-systolic indices which are the most reliable indices of events occurring at the level of the left ventricular muscle fiber, directly reflecting the intrinsic inotropic state without influence of loading conditions.[1,9]

Unlike skeletal muscle, cardiac muscle is not fully activated during contraction.[1] The capacity of the ventricle to augment contractile state to improve overall performance is an important compensatory mechanism in many disease states. Actual quantitation of left ventricular contractile reserve has become possible using either pharmacologic agents (such as dobutamine) or dynamic exercise testing techniques.

To date, data acquired at the time of cardiac catheterization have been used as the "gold standard" for all noninvasive imaging techniques. It has been assumed that any disparity between invasive and echocardiographic findings results from inherent inaccuracies or technical problems with ultrasound imaging. Indeed, there are enough differences between angiographic and cardiac ultrasound methods to raise major questions about the validity of such comparisons.[10,11] These include:

— Angiographic techniques visualize cavity silhouettes while two-dimensional echo-cardiography also gives wall thickness and detailed data on cardiac anatomy.
— Cardiovascular physiology at the time of catheterization may not be representative of the patient's true hemodynamic status due to the volume and pressure effects of contrast materials in the left ventricle.
— Since angiographic contrast material is usually cleared from the left ventricle within three to five beats, only a limited number of hemodynamically stable beats are available for data analysis. With two-dimensional echocardiography, left ventricular performance can be assessed serially in an unlimited number of cardiac cycles.

Cardiac output

Cardiac output measurements are among the most important physiological indices of cardiovascular function. They are used in a wide variety of clinical settings, including operating room, intensive care units, cardiac catheterization laboratories, etc. Cardiac output measurements can help the anesthesiologist assess the clinical status of patients and can assist in determining therapeutic needs and making prognoses. Serial cardiac output measurements help the anesthesiologist evaluate the effectiveness of pharmacologic therapy. Cardiac output measurements are useful in selecting the "best-PEEP" settings for artificial ventilation[12] and, in the case of pacing, optimal pacing rates.[13]

Various approaches to determine cardiac output have been developed but lack of effectiveness has prevented their wide acceptance in clinical medicine. The present method of choice for measuring cardiac output is the thermodilution method, which involves the transvenous insertion of a pulmonary artery catheter. A major disadvantage of this method, apart from its invasivenes,[14] is the requirement for interactive central venous fluid injections to measure cardiac output, which makes continuous measurements impossible. Moreover, erroneous cardiac output values can be obtained by the thermodilution method when large volumes of fluid are being administrated to the right heart, which is common during surgery (cardiopulmonary bypass pump, anhepatic period of liver transplantation, rapid infusion through a large intravenous catheter, etc.). Moreover, one must keep in mind that the thermodilution technique measures right-sided cardiac output. This is important because the technique cannot be used for patients with intracardiac shunts: totally erroneous data will be obtained (left-to-right shunt will show falsely elevated cardiac output).

Thus, an optimal method for monitoring cardiac output, especially when applied to critically ill patients, should allow continuous and noninvasive determination of cardiac output with little need of perfusion interaction. These conditions have been met by TEE in providing two quite different approaches, namely two-dimensional volumes and Doppler aortic or pulmonary flows.[15,16]

Formulas for cardiac output and variables that can be calculated from left ventricular dimensions and volumes are shown in Table 6.1. Stroke volume is the amount of blood ejected from the left ventricle per beat and is a function of the

Table 6.1. Formulas for variables that can be calculated by means of TEE dimensions and volumes

Formula	Normal value range
$SV_{2D} = EDV - ESV$	50–80 ml
$SV_{Doppl} = TVI \times CSA$	60–90 ml
$CO = SV \times HR$	3.6–5.6 l/min
$CI = CO/BSA$	2.0–3.5 l/min/m^2
$EF = (EDV - ESV)/EDV$	0.53–0.64
$FS(\%\Delta D) = (EDD - ESD)/EDD$	0.31–0.38
$EFA = (EDA - ESA)/EDA$	0.51–0.59
$Vcf = [(EDD - ESD)/EDD]/LVET$	1.02–1.94 circ/sec

SV_{2D} stroke volume derived from two-dimensional long axis left ventricular four-chamber plane; SV_{Doppl} stroke volume derived from Doppler aortic or pulmonary flow; *TVI* Doppler determined time-velocity integral; *CSA* cross-sectional area through which Doppler is sampled; *CO* cardiac output; *CI* cardiac index; *EDV* end-diastolic volume; *ESV* end-systolic volume; *EDA* end-diastolic area; *ESA* end-systolic area; *EF* ejection fraction; *FS* (%ΔD) = fractional shortening; *Vcf* mean velocity of circumferential fiber shortening; *EFA* ejection fraction area; *BSA* body surface area.

overall extent of left ventricular fiber shortening. Cardiac output is stroke volume times heart rate. Due to compensatory mechanisms, the dilated or hypertophic left ventricle may still eject a normal or near-normal cardiac output, despite significant depression in contractility.[1] In general, cardiac output indices are dependent upon preload, afterload, heart rate and contractility. Therefore, none of these indices can be used separately as an index for left ventricular contractility.[1,10]

Two-dimensional method

Reliable estimation of cardiac output by the two-dimensional method depends on the proper determination of the left ventricular volumes, which in turn depends on numerous factors. These include adequate imaging of the left ventricular endocardial border, reproducible probe positioning and proper alignment of the imaging plane by obtaining true short- and long-axis tomographic cuts of the ventricle. The formula for calculating cardiac output by two-dimensional echocardiography is:

$$\mathbf{CO = (EDV - ESV) \times HR}$$

where CO = cardiac output; EDV = end-diastolic volume; ESV = end-systolic volume and HR = heart rate. For two-dimensional echocardiographic determination of left ventricular volumes see the chapter on preload.

Both volumes are calculated using one of the methods described earlier (see the chapter on preload). The two-dimensional echocardiographic stroke volume generally shows a better correlation with the comparable angiographic measurement than does the end-diastolic volume but a lower correlation than the end-systolic volume. In absolute terms. the echocardiographic stroke volume appears to be a more accurate estimate of the comparable angiographic volume than are either the end-diastolic or the end-systolic volumes taken by themselves. This increased accuracy occurs because the consistent errors in both volume calculations cancel out when the values are subtracted[17]. Two-dimensional echocardiographic stroke volume has been reported to average $44 \pm 14 \, \text{ml/m}^2$.[18]

In all methods, stroke volume should be determined at end-expiration, because it has been shown that left ventricular stroke volume normally decreased during inspiration.[19]

Because two-dimensional echocardiographic estimation of cardiac output is based on the geometric assumption of chamber size and shape, this method is limited by ventricular asynergy. Moreover, with TEE it may be difficult to obtain a true left ventricular long-axis image, because it may not be technically possible to direct the ultrasound beam through the apex from the confines of the esophagus.[11,20,21] Hence, as a result of foreshortening of the left ventricle and inability to visualize the ventricular apex, exact cardiac output derived from volume measurements will be difficult. More promising is Doppler determination of cardiac output, which expands the utility of TEE in perioperative monitoring.

Doppler echocardiographic method

Theory

As mentioned earlier, assessment of cardiac output using two-dimensional echo-cardiography is based on a geometric assumption of chamber size and shape. In contrast, Doppler echocardiography provides left ventricular output data without the need for geometric assumptions. It measures the *net results* of the pumping action of the left ventricle using principles that are different from those used in anatomic imaging.

By TEE Doppler echocardiographic measurements of cardiac output, blood flow velocity is measured in the aorta by quantitation of the change in frequency between the emitted ultrasonic signal and the signal reflected from red blood cells. This change in frequency (f) is called the Doppler shift, and is related to blood velocity by the Doppler equation

$$V = \frac{c}{2fo} \times \frac{\Delta f}{\cos \theta}$$

where V equals the velocity of blood flow, Δf equals the Doppler frequency shift (which is measured) or the difference between the frequencies of emitted and reflected signals, fo equals the frequency of the emitted ultrasonic signals, c equals the velocity of sound in tissue (approximately 1540 m/sec), and θ equals the angle of incidence between the direction of blood flow and the direction of emitted ultrasonic signal. One can then derive blood flow velocity. From the blood flow velocity, one can subsequently calculate stroke volume. The stroke volume is calculated from the integration of the instantaneous blood flow velocity over the cross-sectional area of the aorta during the time of one cardiac cycle. By multiplying the average stroke volume by the mean heart rate, one arrives at cardiac output.

$$\text{Stroke volume}^{16} = \int_{\substack{\text{Time of} \\ \text{cardiac} \\ \text{cycle}}} \int \int_{\substack{\text{Cross-sectional} \\ \text{area of the} \\ \text{aorta}}} \mathbf{v}(x, y, t) \, \mathcal{f} \, a \, da \, dt$$

The final formula used in the computers of modern sonograph is:

$$\text{Cardiac index}^{8,15} = \text{TVI} \times \text{CSA/BSA} \, (l/\text{min/m}^2)$$

where TVI is the Doppler time velocity integral in cm, i.e., the area under the Doppler curve, which the echocardiographer has to outline; CSA is the cross-sectional area of the interrogated vessel or valve in cm^2; BSA = body surface area in m^2. In practical terms these calculations require:

— An accurate temporal representation of the Doppler blood flow velocity with its maximal value. With all sampling sites for velocity measurements, it is important to optimize the Doppler signal as much as possible. This means minimizing the angle between the direction of the ultrasonic signal and the direction of blood flow, and maximizing signal amplitude. The examination must search out the maximum Doppler shift, using all available aids, using the pitch and intensity of the auditory signal, and the amplitude and gray scale intensity of the spectral display.[8,16] Doppler velocity data are then integrated with respect to time for calculation of the time velocity integral.

—All Doppler techniques require the use of two-dimensional echocardiographic measurement of diameter of the orifice or vessel through which blood flows, for converting to cross-sectional area.

In practice, several Doppler techniques exist for measurement of cardiac output. Although we have discussed the theory behind the measurement of cardiac output at the *aorta*, the continuity equation shows that other sites can also be used to measure cardiac output. The continuity equation states that the flow measured at one cross-sectional area of the tube is equal to the flow measured at another cross-section as long as there is no gain or loss of fluid between the two cross-sections. Thus, we can see that flow at the aortic root (neglecting coronary flow) is equal to flow in the left ventricular outflow tract and inflow through the mitral valve. Similarly, the flow in the main pulmonary artery is the same as in the right ventricular outflow tract and across the tricuspid valve.

Cardiac output by sampling the aortic valve

The best TEE position for sampling the aorta for cardiac output calculation is a modification of the transgastric short-axis view of the mid-left ventricular level to the apical left ventricular level. This can be accomplished by further insertion of the transesophageal probe and anterior flexion of the tip of the probe (Fig. 6.1). The above described modification allows visualization of the left ventricular outflow tract, aortic valve and ascending aorta. Manipulations of the transesophageal probe are made by slight insertion, withdrawal or lateral flexion to align the ultrasound beam as much as possible parallel with the blood flow across the aortic valve.[22,23]

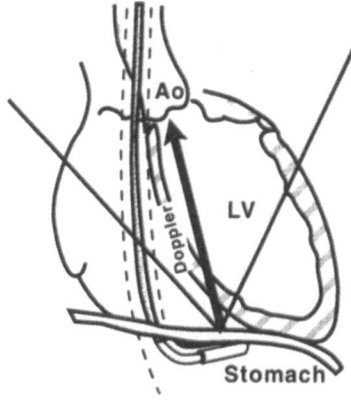

Fig. 6.1. Schematic diagram showing the position of the transesophageal transducer to align the ultrasound beam parallel to blood flow for transgastric Doppler determination of left ventricular cardiac output. Note that the angle between the Doppler beam and the proximal part of the ascending aorta just distal to the aortic valve should be nearly 0°. Two-dimensional echo fan (arc) is given as an angle; *LV* left ventricle; *Ao* aorta

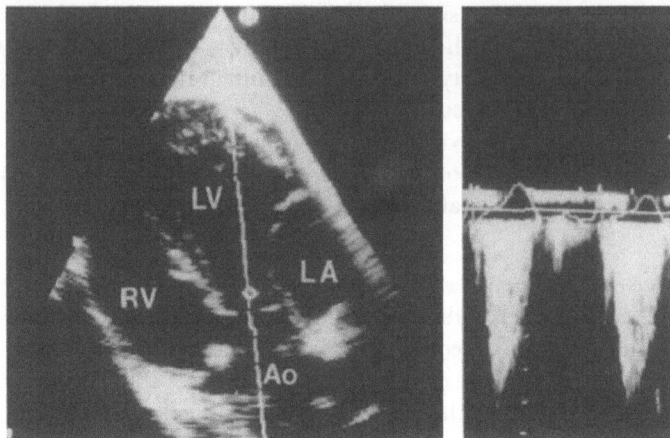

Fig. 6.2. Left: transgastric view of aortic valve and left ventricular outflow tract with continuous wave Doppler cursor aligned parallel to flow in proximal part of ascending aorta. Right: transgastric continuous Doppler spectral display of blood flow across the aortic valve. *LV* left ventricle; *RV* right ventricle; *LA* left atrium; *Ao* aorta

The steerable continuous wave Doppler cursor is then aligned parallel with the flow through the aortic valve (Figs. 6.1 and 6.2). The continuous wave Doppler is preferred because of the Nyquist limit of the pulsed wave Doppler. Pulsed Doppler can also be used for measurements only if the frequency shift is less than 1/2 of the sampling frequency. Color mapping of the left ventricular outflow tract, as proposed by some authors,[23] is unnecessary because both conventional and color Doppler are angle dependent.

The internal systolic aortic valve area is determined best from an esophageal level (mid or high) that images the left ventricular outflow tract and aortic valve (Fig. 6.3). The area through which the blood passes can be calculated by two different methods: (a) area $= \pi \times$ (aortic valve diameter/2)^2, which assumes a circular geometry[22] and (b) *area* $= 0.5 \times \cos 30\cdot \times S^2$, assuming a triangular shape through which the blood is ejected. In the latter formula cross sectional area is calculated as the area of an equilateral triangle,[23] using the TEE frame in which each aortic valve cusp tip appeared as a near straight line describing one side of the triangle (Fig. 6.3). In our experience the first calculation is more rational and gives more correct results.

Cardiac output by sampling the pulmonic valve

The proximal part of the main pulmonary artery above the pulmonic valve is parallel to the Doppler ultrasound beam by TEE in the basal transesophageal plane (Figs. 6.4 and 6.5), which is not difficult for visualizing.[24,25] The pulsed Doppler cursor is then directed parallel to the blood flow as much as possible within the main pulmonary artery, placing the sample volume cursor just above the level of the

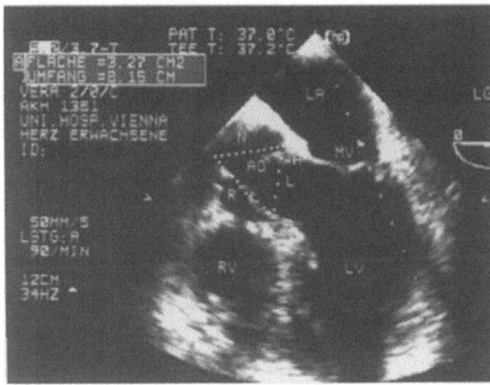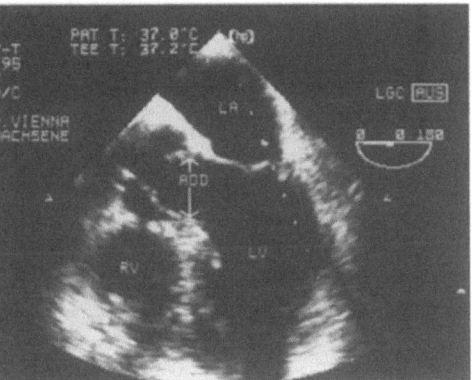

Fig. 6.3. Left: Aortic valve and left venticle with left atrium from midesophageal view during left ventricular ejection (mitral valve is closed and aortic valve is open. One can see the approximately triangular shape of the aortic valve at time of systole. Cusps appear as nearly straight lines. The leaflets' fusion points identify the corners of a equilateral triangle, which allows calculation of the valve area according to the formula: $0.5 \times \cos 30° \times S^2$. Right: From the same image measurement of the aortic valve diameter is shown by calculation of the aortic valve area according to the formula: $\pi \times (\text{aortic valve diameter}/2)^2$. *AO* aortic valve; *N* noncoronary cusp; *L* left coronary cusp; *R* right coronary cusp; *AOD* aortic valve diameter; *MV* mitral valve; *LA* left atrium; *LV* left ventricle; *RV* right ventricle; *S* average length of the three sides of the triangle

pulmonic valve. Slight adjustment of the position and angulation of the transesophageal probe is made to obtain a high-quality Doppler spectral display (Fig. 6.5). Calculation of the valve area is made using the formula area $= \pi \times (\text{pulmonic valve diameter}/2)^2$.

Using this method, the placement of the transducer in the midbasal esophagus appears to be the best location to measure blood flow in the main pulmonary artery, which is directed toward the transducer. However, Doppler pulmonary artery catheter capable of continuous right ventricular cardiac output measurement is not available (but look promising).[25a]

Theoretically, mitral and tricuspid valves can also be sampled for estimation of cardiac output, but because their orifices are not constant throughout diastole[20, 25] the calculations may not be correct. Nevertheless, Doppler transatrioventricular inflows are invaluable for the assessment of ventricular diastolic function.[8, 26]

Fundamental sources of error

As mentioned earlier, three quantities must be measured for the calculation of flow rate, namely, the mean transluminal blood flow velocity, i.e., time velocity integral, the cross-sectional area of the orifice and the angle of incidence. Each of these is associated with a potential error. We have already said that the signal must be maximal. A fundamental problem in the determination of the cross-sectional area is the fact that this area is commonly computed from two-dimensional echocardiography.

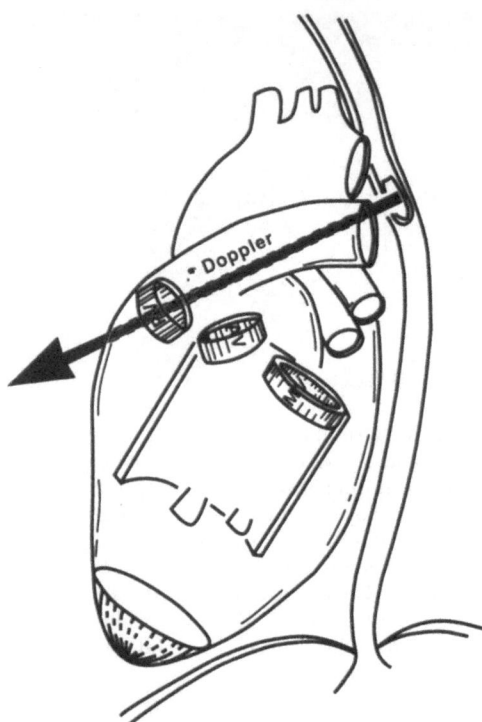

Fig. 6.4. Diagram of the position of the transesophageal transducer to align the ultrasound beam parallel to blood flow for basal esophageal Doppler determination of right ventricular cardiac output. Note that the angle between the Doppler ultrasound beam and the main pulmonary artery should be nearly 0°. *PV* pulmonary valve; *AV* aortic valve, *MV* mitral valve

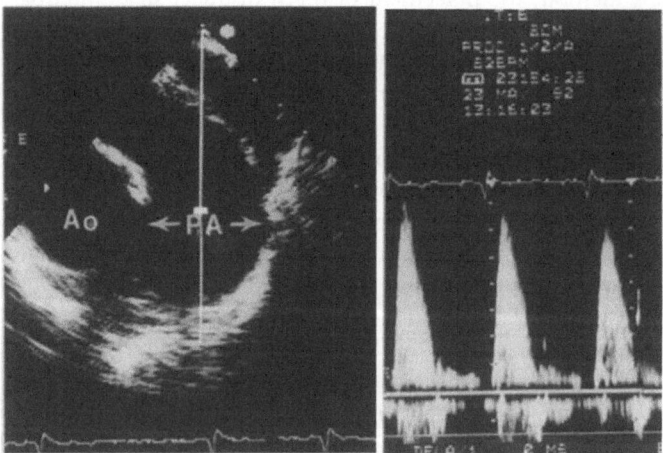

Fig. 6.5. Left: Basal esophageal view of the main pulmonary artery with pulsed wave Doppler cursor aligned parallel to the blood flow in the main pulmonary artery. Right: From the same position Doppler spectral display of blood flow across the pulmonic valve is shown. *PA* main pulmonary artery; *Ao* aorta

By squaring the radius, one squares the error as well. Such an inaccuracy can occur as a consequence of the limited spatial resolution of the ultrasound equipment. A realistic assumption is that the error is between 10 and 20%.

An angle θ parallel to flow will produce the greatest Doppler time velocity integral $(\cos 0 = 1)$. The Doppler beam must be directed as much as possible parallel to flow (less than 15·); otherwise the angle of correction must be calculated.[15] Doppler measurements of cardiac output require a long period of training and often a long time is required to obtain a satisfactory signal.[27]

Comparison with other methods of cardiac measurement

Many studies have been undertaken to compare Doppler cardiac output measurements with other flow measurements, including experiments in vitro and in vivo; in humans and in animals; using green dye, thermodilution and Fick techniques.[24] The findings may be summarized and generalized as follows:

— The best sampling position for TEE Doppler estimation of cardiac output is the aortic valve, which gives very good correlation with invasive techniques;[22,23] second best is the pulmonic valve, which also shows a good correlation with invasive standards.[21]
— Correlation with Doppler is often better with in vitro techniques than in vivo comparison with thermodilution. Schuster and Nanda[16] concluded that this is in part due to the weakness of thermodilution as a "gold standard," in addition to the innate limitations of the Doppler technique.

Uses of Doppler cardiac output in anesthesiology

Evidence exists that the Doppler method is superior to thermodilution techniques.[22–25,27–32] It is well known that thermodilution may be relatively inaccurate.[33] The computation constant takes into account the catheter dead space, injection rate, and the heat change in transit, but there are many other factors that could account for an intrinsic error of thermodilution of at least 10%,[25,34] including volume of injectate, change in catheter position, or inadequate temperature difference between the body and injectate. Haude et al.[31] reported continuous beat-to-beat measure- ment of cardiac output during surgery and in intubated patients in the ICU with a modified TEE probe. They concluded that it is reliable, an "ideal" tool for undertaking hemodynamic studies when continuous monitoring of cardiac output is required, and added that compared with invasive methods, it can be accomplished with little need for personal interaction.

Ejection fraction

The use of ejection fraction , the ratio of the stroke volume to ventricular end-diastolic volume, is well accepted as a clinically useful, quantitative measurement of ventricular performance.[35] One may ask why the normal ejection fraction remains at a value of 0.5–0.6 rather than, for example, 0.1 to 0.9. Teleologic and cardiac physiologic reasoning would suggest that there must be an advantage, on the one hand, in terms of efficient energy utilization; on the other hand, coronary flow occurs mostly in early diastole (see the chapter on ischemia).

Using the Frank-Starling functional curves the lowest ejection fraction would be associated with a high afterload, low preload, and minimal intrinsic contractility. Hence, improvement of ejection fraction can be obtained by reducing afterload, increasing preload or augmenting intrinsic contractility, depending on the position of the curve (see section on contractility). Because of the extremely high load dependence of ejection fraction and the large number of ways through which the cardiovascular system, by changes in ejection fraction, may alter arterial and venous resistance and compliance, ejection fraction seems not to measure ventricular performance, but "integrated system" performance. Ejection fraction appears to be an efficient and integrated measure of the entire cardiovascular system's ability to cope with abnormalities in any or all of the three critical variables (preload, afterload and contractility) that determine ventricular performance.

The use of ejection fraction to evaluate left ventricular function has become common in everyday anesthesia practice with the introduction of automated boundary detection systems (Hewlett Packard, Andover, MA), which display instantly beat-to-beat values of this parameter. Moreover, the addition of Doppler flow determination to the same transducer head allows concurrent evaluation of valvular competence necessary to correctly interpret ejection fraction, because either mitral or aortic valvular incompetence can lead to an increase in ejection fraction that may be falsely interpreted and reflect normal ventricular function.[36]

Although the measurement of left ventricular systolic performance by ejection fraction is adequate for a gross assessment of overall pump function, it is unable to separate changes in left ventricular contractility from alterations in other determinants of left ventricular fiber shortening (i.e., preload, afterload and heart rate). As such, left ventricular ejection fraction reflects a complex interaction between ventricular loading conditions and contractile state.[37,38] For example, in the normal heart, an increase in left ventricular afterload is associated with an increase in end-diastolic volume, with maintainence of stroke volume. If the increase in left ventricular afterload becomes excessive for a given level of contractility, the rise in end-diastolic volume may exceed the ventricle's ability to augment end-diastolic volume, resulting in a fall in stroke volume.[1] This is known as exhaustion of preload reserve, and reflects a mismatch between afterload, preload and contractility. The net result is a fall in ventricular ejection fraction despite stable left ventricular contractility. This is a frequent occurrence in patients with a dilated ventricle. Other examples of conditions in which EF can give misleading data regarding intrinsic left ventricular contractile properties include decreased intravascular volume (hypovolemia), hypertension, response to cardioactive pharmacologic agents and left heart valvular lesions.[1] It becomes readily apparent that during rapid changes of left ventricular loading conditions, as in surgical procedures or use of vasoactive drugs, left ventricular ejection fraction must be interpreted cautiously as a nonspecific parameter.

Nevertheless, with reasonable clinical judgment, the use of left ventricular ejection fraction has become established as a good clinical estimate of left ventricular function, most convincingly in the anesthetic preoperative[37,39] as well as intraoperative evaluation of patients.[40–44]

Because technologic advances allowing automated left ventricular end-systolic pressure-volume relation (the best intrinsic contractility parameter) are not thus far easily applicable, ejection fraction will continue to be the single and most commonly used clinical quantitative measurement of ventricular pump performance. Moreover, very good correlation coefficient between angiographic and two-dimensional echocardiographic estimated ejection fraction have been reported ($r = 0.83$, using prolate ellipsoid model[45] and $r = 0.98$ using Simpson's rule[46]).

Practical remarks on measurement of ejection fraction

— Right and left ventricular ejection fraction must be estimated using midesophageal four-chamber plane with biventricular long-axis view, based on measuring end-diasdtolic and end-systolic volumes, as described in chapter preload.
— Outlining end-diastolic and end-systolic ventricular contours should be done by means of leading edge-leading edge method (see the chapter on preload).
— Tricuspidal and mitral rings must be measured from the inner edge of the lateral right corner of the annulus to the inner edge of the medial corner just below insertion of the leaflets; they make complicated spatial movements during contraction (Fig. 6.6).
— A common source of error in ejection fraction measurement is respiration.

Inspiration decreases the intrathoracic pressure, causing an increase in systemic venous return and in right ventricular volume, which itself reduces left ventricular end-diastolic volume via diastolic ventricular interdependence.[45] In addition, inspiration increases the left ventricular afterload, thus, reducing the left ventricular stroke volume. The different mechanisms combine to produce a decrease in end-diastolic left ventricular dimensions, with no change in end-systolic dimensions and a decrease in stroke volume and ejection fraction. Beat-to-beat variability at end-expiration in the measurement of ejection fraction is significantly less than during inspiration[19]. Therefore, as mentioned earlier, measurements should be taken during end-expiration. Simultaneous recording of respiration facilitates analysis of echocardiographic images at end-expiration and provides a more reliable assessment of left ventricular function.

Fractional shortening and percent area of change. These parameter are equivalent to ejection fraction; the difference is that left ventricular dimensions are used instead of volumes (Table 6.1). They have the same clinical limitations as discussed for ejection fraction.

In past the fractional shortening, %ΔD, has been derived from M-mode recording and rely on minor axis shortening as a representation of overall ventricular systolic function. It is based on the angiographic observation that the

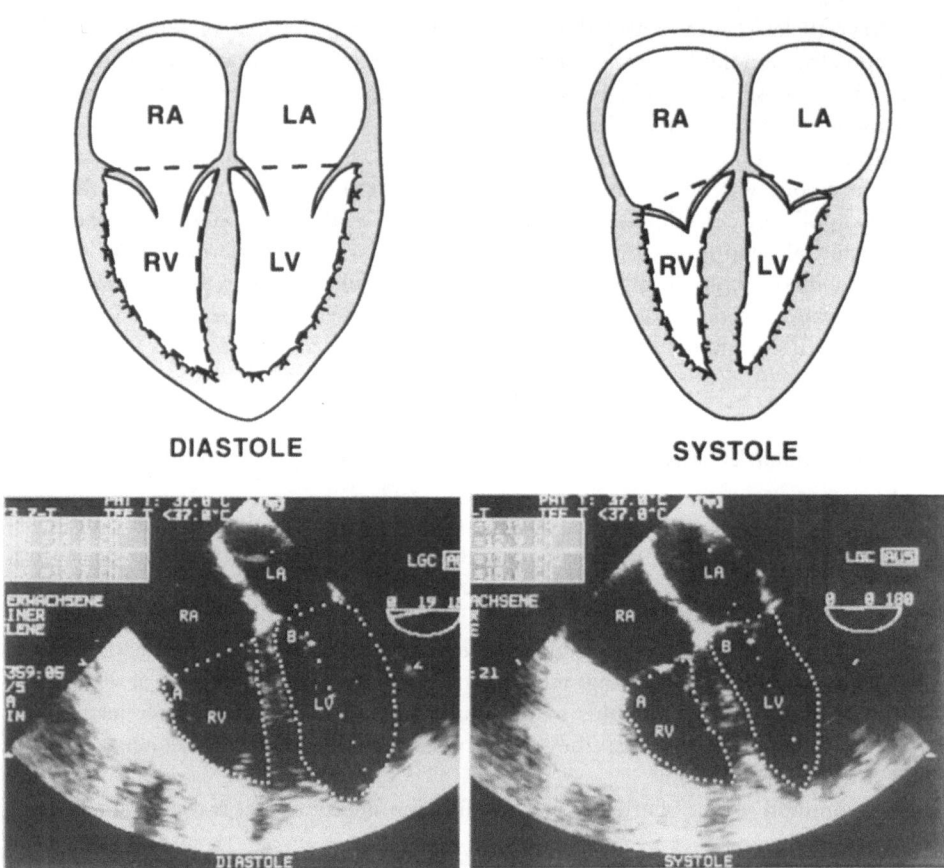

Fig. 6.6. Midesophageal four-chamber plane with biventricular long-axis view for measurement of ejection fraction. *RA* right atrium; *LA* left atrium; *RV* right ventricle; *LV* left ventricle

systolic decrease in ventricular volume is primarily due to minor axis shortening and that the percentage of changes in the minor axis during systole shows a linear correlation with ejection fraction.[48] Unfortunately, although the simplicity of this method is attractive, it has major limitations. The most important limitation is that the method seeks to define left ventricular size and function from a single arbitrarily dimension and consequently must assume that the recorded measurement actually corresponds to the one of the minor axes of the ellipsoid model and that the function of the ventricle in the region in which the dimension is taken is representative of global ventricular function. There are important exceptions to both of these assumption. In ischemic heart disease, e.g., major local abnormalities in left ventricular structures and function may be present in areas of the left ventricle that are removed from the sampled region.

In the symmetrically contracting ventricle fractional shortening (FS) represents a simple method for estimating ventricular function and can be calculated from the left ventricular internal dimension using the following formula:[10,11]

$$\%\Delta D \text{ or } FS = \frac{Dd - Ds}{Dd} \times 100$$

In patients with normal left ventricular function, $\%\Delta D$ is usually greater than 25%.

To overcome partly the limitation of the above mentioned $\%\Delta D$ calculation, two-dimensional cavity area, A_c, can be planimetered to express an area change. Alternatively, the area can be converted into a mean ventricular diameter, and D can be expressed as:

$$D = 2 \times \sqrt{(A_c/\pi)}$$

Such a method, with A_c measured at the papillary muscles level in the two-dimensional short-axis view, provides smaller normal values for shortening thanM-mode measurements ($30 \pm 5\%$ vs $35 \pm 5\%$, our unpublished data).

Unfortunately, major changes in left ventricular morphology often appear near the apex and remain unaccounted for by the fractional shortening approach.

Mean velocity of circumferential fiber shortening (Vcf)

This measures the mean velocity of ventricular fiber shortening at the level of the left ventricular minor axis.[5,10] It is calculated as the percent fractional shortening divided by the left ventricular ejection time (see also Table 6.1).

Vcf = [(EDD − ESD)/EDD]/LVET

where EDD is left ventricular end-diastolic dimension; ESD is left ventricular end-systolic dimension and LVET denotes left ventricular ejection time, which can be measured from aortic Doppler display (Figs. 6.7, 6.8) or from the noninvasive external carotid pulse tracing (invasive arterial pressure record, respectively); in the latter case by measuring the time interval between the upstroke of the arterial pulse to the incisura. The value of Vcf is expressed in circumferences per second (circ/sec). This value is normalized for end-diastolic chamber size, and therefore is useful for comparisons between patients. Mean velocity of circumferential fiber shortening is misnamed; in reality Vcf represents the velocity of the shortening of the minor axis and not of the whole circumference. It does not reflect the change in geometry during contraction or regional wall motion abnormality. This consideration does not minimize the usefulness of Vcf but pinpoints one of the limitations.

Vcf is relatively preload-independent. However, it is highly afterload-, contractility-, and heart rate-dependent. A Vcf value corrected for heart rate (Vcf_c) has been clinically useful when plotted against ventricular afterload.[5] Rate-corrected Vcf is calculated by multiplying Vcf by the square root of the preceding R–R interval, obtained from the electrocardiogram.

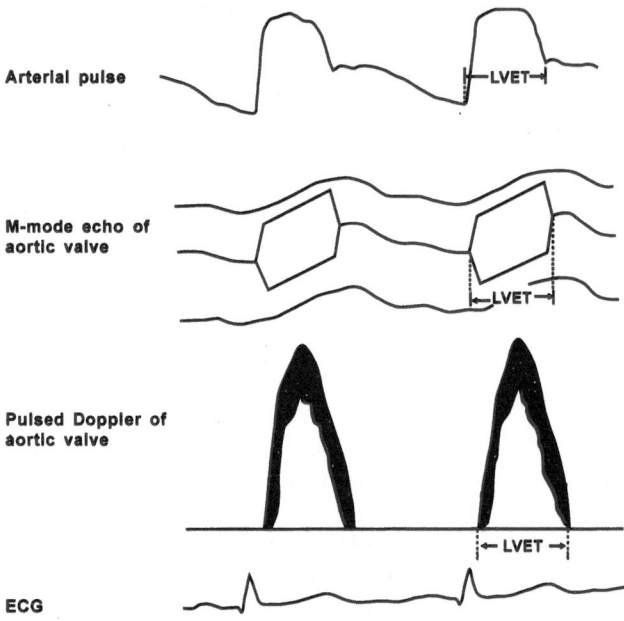

Fig. 6.7. Left ventricular ejection time (LVET) can be measured using three methods, including 1) arterial pressure curve; 2) M-mode echocardiogram of the aortic valve; and 3) pulsed Doppler recording from aortic valve and proximal aorta

Two-dimensional Doppler echocardiographic estimation of isovolumic phase indexes

Peak positive rate of change of left ventricular pressure (dP/dt)

The isovolumic indices of left ventricular performance are determined from pressure transients recorded during the period between closure of the mitral valve and opening of the aortic valve (Fig. 6.8). The most commonly used isovolumic index is the maximal rate of left ventricular pressure rise (i.e., peak positive dP/dt). It is derived by electronic differentiation of the left ventricular pressure curve[49] and is also called the first derivative of left ventricular pressure. In physical terms, the basic curve (pressure) represents the path, and its first derivative (dP/dt) gives the speed at the different points in this path.[49] Decreased values represent depressed myocardial contractility.

If mitral regurgitation is present (not rare in patients with ischemic heart diseases), noninvasive evaluation of dP/dt is possible by Doppler echocardiography.

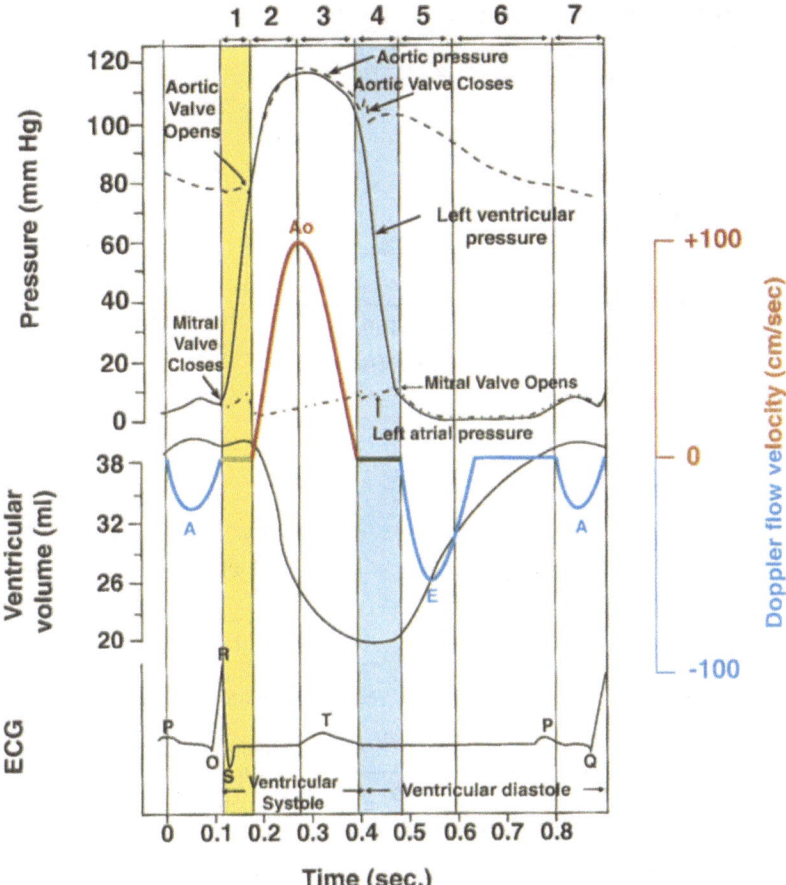

Fig. 6.8. Classical schematic representation of the time intervals or phases of the cardiac cycle by means of aortic pressure curve, left ventricular pressure curve, left atrial pressure with Doppler aortic and mitral flows. *1* isovolumic contraction phase; *2* rapid ejection phase; *3* late (reduced) ejection phase; *4* isovolumic relaxation phase; *5* rapid ventricular filling; *6* slow (reduced) ventricular filling or diastasis; *7* atrial systole, i.e., atrial contribution to ventricular filling. Note that the beginning and the end of isovolumic phases are determined by a crossover of two invasive pressure curves as well as by a beginning and end of Doppler flow velocity curves. *Ao* Doppler aortic flow; *E* early diastolic mitral peak filling rate; *A* atrial diastolic peak filling

The complete velocity profile of regurgitant flow through the mitral valve can be recorded by continuous wave Doppler echocardiography. Using the simplified Bernoulli equation, the velocity curve can be converted to a pressure gradient ΔP ($\Delta P = 4V^2$, where ΔP is the pressure gradient in millimeters mercury and V is the instantaneous regurgitant jet velocity in meters per second) curve, the derivative of which gives instantaneous $d\Delta P/dt$ (Fig. 6.9). From this measurement peak $d\Delta P/dt$

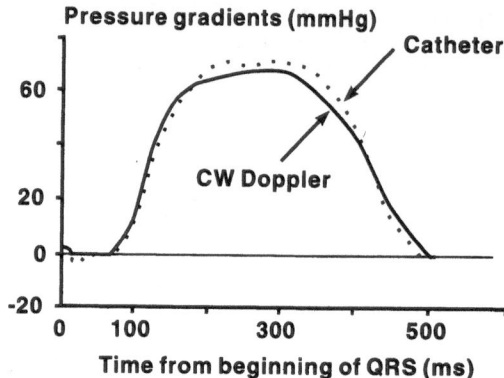

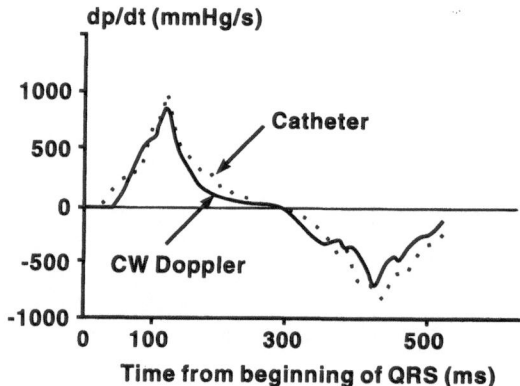

Fig. 6.9. Top: Graph comparing Doppler derived left ventriculo-atrial pressure gradient curve with gradient curve derived from cather-recorded simultaneous left atrial and left ventricular pressures. Bottom: Graph comparing dP/dt curve determined by Doppler mitral regurgitant velocity spectrum with dP/dt curve derived from catheter-recorded left ventricular pressure curve

has an excellent correlation with invasive measurements $(r = 0.97)^{50}$ The main limitations of Doppler dΔP/dt method are: (a) mitral regurgitation must be present, which is not the case in all patients; (b) early diastole is not truly isovolumic, because of mitral insufficiency. The latter concern, however, has not been a significant problem in the experimental settings.

Isovolumic contraction time (IVCT)

Similarly to mechanocardiography, using Doppler recordings one can estimate the duration of isovolumic contraction time, i.e., the time at the beginning of left ventricular contraction when both mitral and aortic valves are closed (Fig. 6.8). It is expressed in msec (normal value 75 ± 18 msec), or some prefer the ratio IVCT/ ejection time, because a ratio does not need correction for heart rate and perhaps is less sensitive to preload.[8] Nevertheless, despite normalization of dP/dt and IVCT, they are not independent from loading conditions.

Frank-Starling principle and end-systolic ventricular performance curves

Quantification of load independent noninvasive contractile indices, reflecting the true inotropic state of the myocardium, remains a challenge in practical cardiology. All traditional indices described in the first section of this chapter are highly load-dependent, and thus, reflect overall left ventricular performance rather than contractility (Table 6.2).

Frank and Starling established a relationship between isovolumic peak pressure and volume during the active state in the intact frog heart. It was that "Increased diastolic distension exercises a strong augmenting effect on ventricular contraction." This ultimately became known as the Frank-Starling law of the heart. Neither Frank nor Starling demonstrated any modulation of the pressure-volume curves by afterload or inotropy, and, for some time after their work was published, the regulation of cardiac output was thought to be effected entirely by the Frank-Starling mechanism.

But although the Frank-Starling mechanism is important in denervated heart, it is less important in innervated heart under conditions of changing heart rate and afterloads.[51] It is also difficult to study isovolumic contraction directly in the intact human heart, with the complications that arise from the interaction between the autonomic nervous system, the systolic load and ventricular performance. For example, one such Frank-Starling curve, the plot of stroke volume against end-diastolic volume or end-diastolic ventricular area, has for it slope the ejection fraction (Fig. 6.10). Because ejection fraction, defined as the stroke volume divided by the end-diastolic volume, is one means of measuring the slope of the Frank-Starling relationship, the ejection fraction can be used as an indicator of ventricular

Table 6.2. Effects of determinants of overall left ventricular performance on commonly used echcardiographically obtained ejection phase and isovolumic phase indices

	CO	EF	FS	Vcf	Vcf$_c$	dP/dt IVCT
Preload	+	+	+	NC	NC	+
Afterload	+	+	+	+	+	+
Heart rate	+ +	+ /NC	+ /NC	+	NC	+
Contractility	+	+	+	+	+	+ +

Cardiac output cardiac output; *dP/dt* first derivative of ventricular pressure; *EF* ejection fraction; *FS* fractional shortening; *NC* no change; *IVCT* isovolumic contraction time; *Vcf* mean velocity of fiber shortening; *Vcf$_c$* mean velocity of fiber shortening corrected for heart rate.

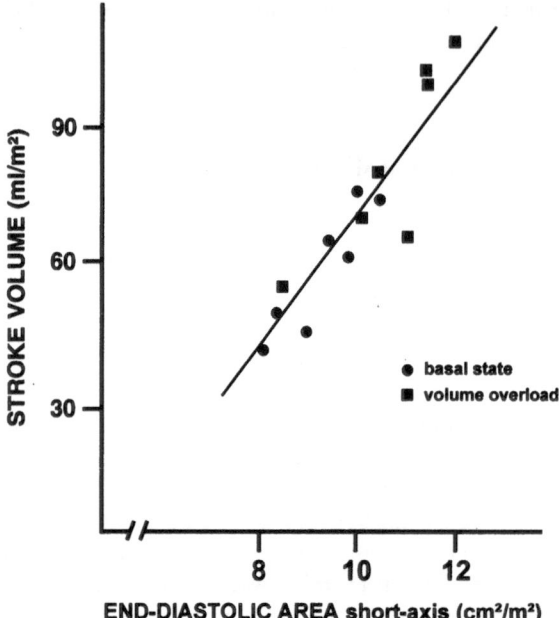

Fig. 6.10. Left ventricular stroke volume index obtained by TEE Doppler sampling of the aorta plotted against TEE left ventricular short-axis end-diastolic area in patients undergoing renal transplantation before and during the time of maximal hydration. Movement along a single curve represents the operation of the Frank-Starling principle, which indicates that stroke volume varies with changes in preload. Upward and to the left or downward and to the right displacement of the curve should represent an augmentation or depression of contractility, respectively (unpublished data)

performance. An important limitation to use the ejection fraction or Frank-Starling relationship for measuring ventricular performance is the inability to account for changes due to afterload and heart rate. Acute changes in systemic arterial pressure that acutely alter afterload on the myocardium are known to alter ejection fraction.[1,52] In theory, according to Frank-Starling relation an increase in end-diastolic pressure, dimension, or volume results in an increase in muscle fiber length. However, these changes in diastolic measurements do not bear a predictable relation to *diastolic* wall stress (i.e., presumed measure of true preload) or to sarcomere length.[1] In addition, factors such as cardiac hypertrophy, pericarditis, and pleural pressure can alter the Frank-Starling relation in the absence of derangements in left ventricular contractile state.[1] In effect, the Frank-Starling relation represents a combination of preload and afterload effects in conjunction with a constant or changing contractile state.

The limitations of the relationship between stroke volume and diastolic volume have led examinations of the relationship between end-systolic pressure and volume as a possible way of incorporating myocardial geometry and loadings into an overall assessment of the contractile state of the left ventricle. These relationships are amongst the most elegant ways of looking at the left ventricular performance, and are conceptually based on the pressure-volume loop (Fig. 6.11).[52] During diastole, the ventricle fills along its exponential passive pressure-volume relation curve, assisted in late diastole by atrial contraction: the time point of the pressure-volume loop moves from end-systolic volume to the end-diastolic volume and pressure that represents preload. During isovolumic force generation, the time point moves vertically upwards from the end-diastolic point. The aortic valve opens when

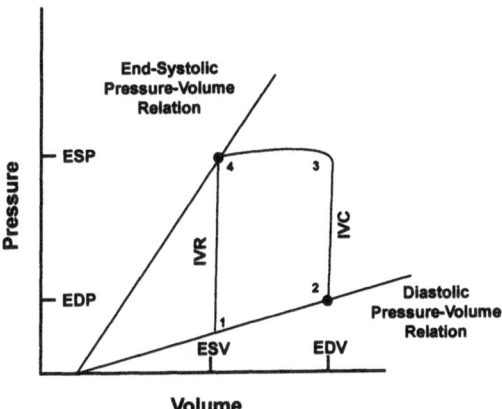

Fig. 6.11. Pressure-volume relationships. Mitral valve opening (point *1*) initiates ventricular filling, marked by leftward progress of the curve, which than reaches to end-diastolic volume point. Point *2* is the mitral valve closure or the end of diastolic pressure-volume line, with subsequent vertical ascending section of the loop indicating the onset of systolic isovolumic contraction (IVC) until point *3* (aortic valve opening). The curve progresses leftward as the aortic valve opens and the ventricle confronts afterload. Ejection concludes at point *4*, i.e., the end-systolic pressure-volume point, which reflect contractility and afterload as well as preload. The curve falls vertically as the isovolumic relaxation (IVR) period of diastole commences. *EDP* end-diastolic pressure; *EDV* end-diastolic volume; *ESP* end-systolic pressure; *ESV* end-systolic volume

the left ventricular pressure exceeds diastolic arterial pressure, the left ventricle confronts its afterload and its volume decreases as the stroke volume is ejected: the time point moves predominately to the left while the pressure rises from approximately arterial diastolic to systolic, and than falls again. When the left ventricular pressure falls below arterial pressure, the aortic valve closes (this time corresponds exactly to the end-systolic arterial pressure; see Fig. 5.6), and the left ventricle relaxes isovolumically; the time point falls vertically at end-systolic volume from the active (systolic) to the passive (diastolic) pressure-volume relationship. When left ventricular pressure falls below left atrial pressure, the mitral valve opens and diastolic filling begins again.

The reason that the pressure-volume loop has gained recent favor as a descriptor of ventricular performance is related to studies of Shuga and Sagawa[53] which latter have been confirmed by others.[9] They obtained a series of isovolumic contractions from a number of different end-diastolic volumes by clamping the aorta in an isolated heart so that the left ventricle could not eject blood. The plot of peak pressure against chamber volume made a fairly strait line that was termed the isovolumic pressure-volume line for the current degree of inotropy (Fig. 6.12). It represents the active state of the left ventricular muscle fibers. Shuga et al. next allowed the heart to contract normally, using different preloads and afterloads, and recorded pressure-volume loops as illustrated schematically in Fig. 6.13. With the different loading conditions, the top left-hand corners of the pressure-volume loops (which included the end-systolic pressure-volume points) all tended to fall on the

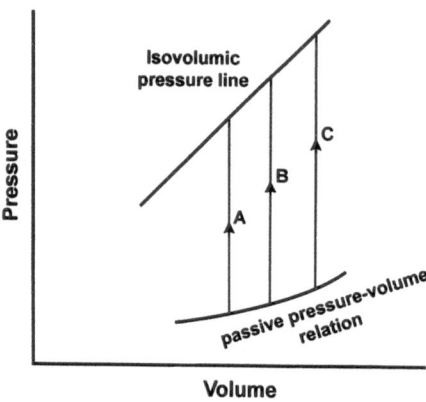

Fig. 6.12. Three isovolumic contractions (*A*, *B*, and *C*) obtained in an isolated dog heart with clamping of the aorta to prevent ejection. The heart contracts isovolumically up to a point and than relaxes along the same line, back to the passive (diastolic) pressure-volume relation. The peak of each contraction defines a line that has been termed the isovolumic pressure line

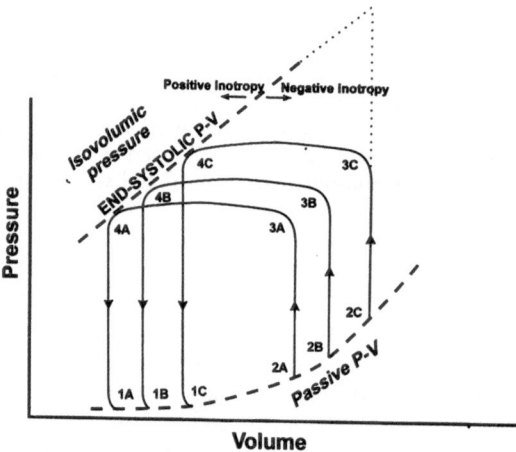

Fig. 6.13. Three pressure-volume loops (*A*, *B*, and *C*) obtained at different pre- and afterloads. The upper left corner of each loop ends on the isovolumic pressure line. This upper left point represents end-systolic pressure (dicrotic notch aortic pressure) and end-systolic volume, thus, forms *end-systolic pressure-volume curve*. Down is shown diastolic (passive) pressure-volume curve. Changes states of inotropy are shown with arrows. *1* opening of the mitral valve; *2* closure of the mitral valve; *3* opening of the aortic valve; *4* closure of the aortic valve; *P–V* ventricular pressure-volume relation

isovolumic pressure-volume line regardless of the preload and afterload. It is important to note that if ejection and therefore reduction in ventricular volume had been prevented, the pressure would have continued rising to a point higher on the same isovolumic pressure-volume line (see dotted line), just as did in Fig. 6.12. The diastolic part of the loop followed the passive pressure-volume relationship. Different states of inotropy were reflected in changes in the slopes of the end-systolic pressure-volume line. Moreover, the intercept of end-systolic pressure-volume lines with the volume axis tended to remain unchanged with changes in inotropy.

The fundamental principle underlying the end-systolic ventricular function curves is that, for any given level of contractility, the end-systolic pressure is proportional (according to the LaPlace law) to the active systolic tension in the myocardial fibers, which depends on fiber length, divided by some function of the ventricular diameters, which is *also* proportional to fiber length. The end-systolic pressure-volume point represent a transient solution to these mathematical relationships between force and geometry at end of the active state, just before relaxation begins.[1,54] The left ventricle contracts to the volume and pressure that can be supported by the length of its contracting fibers.[52]

Because a precise indication of ventricular volume can now be obtained during anesthesia by TEE, there have been numerous efforts to determine end-systolic pressure-volume relationship noninvasively. Thus left ventricular end-systolic pressure is red as end-systolic arterial pressure (see section on afterload; Fig. 5.6), and end-systolic volume is represented by the Simpson's rule method, area or short-axis diameter of the left ventricle as obtained by two-dimensional echocardiography (see section on preload). Attempts to simplify data acquisition by substituting peak systolic pressure for end-systolic pressure, or by using a resting end-systolic pressure to dimension (or volume) ratio are complicated by numerous theoretical as well as physiologic problems.

If a series of pressure-volume points can be obtained under different conditions of preload and afterload, linear least squares regression of volume and pressure will give the slope and intercept of a subject's end-systolic pressure-volume line at a particular state of inotropy.[52] Several significant studies of left ventricular pressure-volume relations have been published by joint anesthesia-cardiology research groups.[2-4,6,55] They plotted end-systolic dimension or end-systolic area on an abscissa x and end-systolic pressure on an ordinate y. Briefly, simple linear regression least-squares method was used to fit each subject's data into a pressure-volume $(P_{ES} = mV_{ES} + b)$ equation, where P_{ES} = end-systolic pressure, V_{ES} = end-systolic volume, m = slope and b = y-intercept.[2-4] The steepness of the slope of the $P_{ES}-V_{ES}$ relation should be directly related to left ventricular contractile state.

There are several problems, however, that need to be emphasized. First of all, it is not precisely clear how one patient can be compared with another. For example, patients with different cardiac sizes will have different end-diastolic volumes. It is intuitive, that one would have to normalize in some way for left ventricular volume. Whether this is best done by expressing volume in terms of body surface area or other means is not clear at this time. Furthermore, with similar baseline contractile properties, left ventricles of different patients will develop different pressures. For example, patient with hypertension or aortic stenosis will develop much higher left ventricular systolic pressures than the patient with normal arterial pressure. In the compensate state, where the intrinsic contractility of the left ventricle is the same, the isovolumic pressure line will be shifted upward in patients with higher ventricular pressures. It is intuitively apparent, therefore, that one must in some way normalize the pressure axis. Some attempts at normalizing have used wall stress on the vertical axis: this may more nearly yield a measurement that can used to compare different patients. O'Kelly et al.[2] have used two-dimensional TEE and end-systolic arterial pressure so as to derive perioperative relationship between end-systolic wall stress and end-systolic chamber area: these showed statistically significant improvement in intrinsic contractility after coronary revascularization. Figure 6.14 illustrates relationship of left ventricular end-systolic wall stress to end-systolic area in patient during orthotopic liver transplantation before and after graft reperfusion demonstrating a depressed cardiac contractility as judged by the slopes of the ventricular function curves.

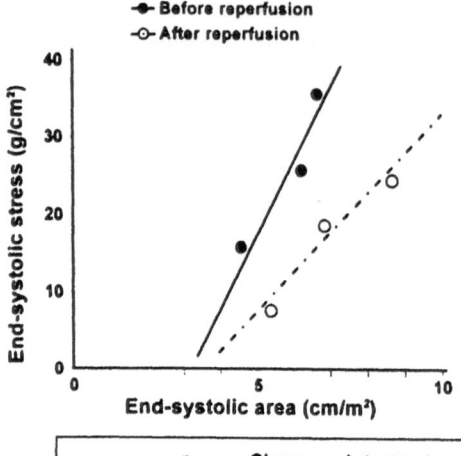

Fig. 6.14. Relationship end-systolic wall stress to TEE estimated left ventricular short-axis end-systolic area in patient during liver transplantation before and 8 min after graft reperfusion according to the equation: Wall stress$_{ES}$ = m Ventricular area$_{ES}$ + b. One can see the right and downward shift of the end-systolic relationship at time of early graft reperfusion consistent with depressed myocardial contractility (unpublished data)

	r	Slope (m)	Intercept
●	0.91	9.2	3.3
○	0.92	3.1	3.5

Other authors have successfully used the relationship of end-systolic wall stress to Vcf (mean velocity of fiber shortening)[5,6] when investigating the effect of different drugs and anesthetic agents on myocardial contractility in the operating room.

Recently, Gorcsan et al.[56] using automatic border detection (Hewlett Packard, Andover, MA) of left ventricular short-axis area and femoral arterial pressure, reported on-line rapid estimation of end-systolic function curves. Femoral arterial pressure, left ventricular cavity area, and electrocardiographic (lead II) signals were simultaneously digitized and recorded on the workstation (computer graphics workstation DN 3550 Apollo Computer, Chelmsford, MA) at a sampling rate of 150 Hz for display. Data were analyzed by automated method, a customized software program written for the same computer workstation used for data acquisition. The program made rapid analysis by automating the pressure and the area waveform alignment by identifying and separating each cardiac cycle by the R wave of the electrocardiogram. Minimum arterial pressure values were automatically aligned with the first occurrence of maximal area values to approximate simultaneous end-diastolic events for each cardiac cycle. Pressure-area loops were than plotted and end-systolic points determined as the maximal pressure/area points. This automated method have allowed for rapid determination of slopes of the end-systolic pressure-volume relations in the operating room by automatic waveform alignment and calculation within 3 sec. Figure 6.15 showed such pressure-volume loops with end-systolic lines before and after cardiopulmonary bypass in patient undergoing coronary artery bypass surgery. For comparison are given simultaneously obtained both left ventricular pressure-volume loops and arterial pressure-volume loops. It is evident that femoral arterial pressure can serve as a surrogate for left ventricular pressure. Further, comparing before and immedi-

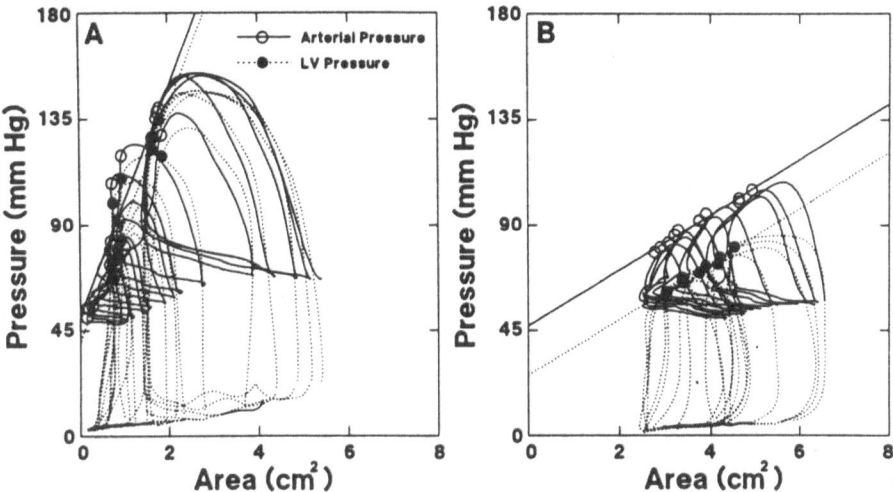

Fig. 6.15. Examples of simultaneous on-line rapid estimated arterial pressure-area loops (solid lines) and ventricular pressure-area loops (dashed lines) before (A) and immediately after (B) cardiopulmonary bypass from the same patient. (From Gorcsan J et al.: Anesthesiology 81:553–562, 1994. Used by permission)

ately after cardiopulmonary bypass there are shift of end-systolic lines to the right and downward.[56]

Although the above mentioned methods have been validated in humans, they have not been widely used in clinical practice, which is mainly due to they complexity: at least two-dimension values, measured at different pressures, are needed to reconstruct the pressure-dimension slope. Thus, determination of the slope for contractility measurements requires transient manipulation of afterload which is sometimes not possible or perhaps even dangerous. A possible alternative to the application of the regression line is to use the quotient between the end-systolic diameter and end-systolic pressure.[57] For one single pressure-volume ratio determination to accurately define the slope of the pressure-volume relation, however, it is necessary to assume that the pressure-volume line runs the origin of the pressure and volume axes (i.e., 0 point of abscissa x and 0 point of ordinate y). Since this is usually not the case[58] the clinical and physiological utility of this index is severely impaired.

Pressure-volume relation can allow a precise administration of vasoactive and inotropic agents (Fig. 6.16).[59] For example, in patients with severe pump (i.e., inotropic) failure, pump function improves after the use of inotropic agents only if there is a contractile reserve. If the myocardial contractile reserve is exhausted or patients are in a state of refractory heart insufficiency, a phosphodiesterase inhibitor, should be considered (reducing afterload and improving myocardial stiffness). Biventricular failure may require a preload increase combined with an afterload decrease.[59]

**End-Systolic Pressure
(or wall stress)**

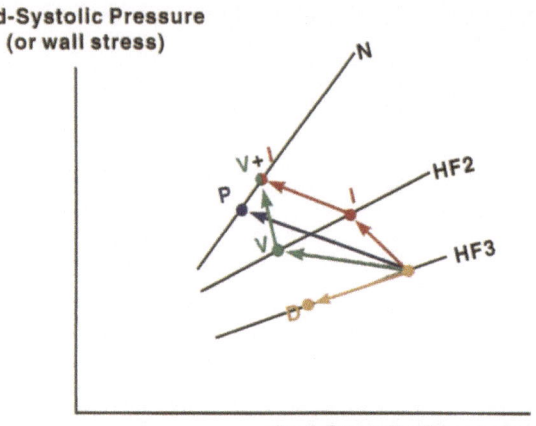

**End-Systolic Dimension
(or Area, Volume, Vcf)**

Fig. 6.16. End-systolic pressure-volume function curves demonstrating modification of left ventricular performance in patients with heart failure and after drug therapy, and hence, the possibility of guiding the therapy. *D* diuretics; *N* normal; *HF2* heart failure grade 2; *HF3* heart failure grade 3; *I* inotropes; *P* phosphodiesterase inhibitors; *V* vasodilators; *Vcf* mean velocity of fiber shortening; *V + I* combination of vasodilators and inotropes

In conclusion, sophisticated end-systolic indices of left ventricular function provide interesting insights into the mechanisms of cardiac performance. They have been useful to assess different interventions in research. In clinical practice, assessment of systolic function generally relies on simpler indices, mainly ejection fraction. With future technological improvements,[56] automated assessment of end-systolic curves are likely to become an everyday clinical reality.

References

1. Braunwald E, Sonnenblick EH, Ross J Jr. Mechanism of cardiac contraction and relaxation. In: Braunwald E, ed, Heart Disease. 4th ed. WB Saunders, Philadelphia, London, pp 351–392, 1992
2. O'Kelly BF, Tubau JF, Knight AA, London MJ, Verrier ED, Mangano DT. Measurement of left ventricular contractility using transesophageal echocardiography in patients undergoing coronary artery bypass grafting. Am Heart J 122: 1041–1049, 1991
3. Mulier JP, Vouters PF, Van Aken H, Vermaut G, Vandermeersch E. Cardiodynamic effects of propofol in comparison with thiopental: Assessment with a transesophageal echocardiographic approach. Anesth Analg 72: 28–35, 1991
4. Heinrich H, Fontaine L, Fösel T, Spilker D, Winter H, Ahnefeld FW. Vergleichende echocardiographische Untersuchungen zur negativen Inotropien von Halothan, Enfluran and Isofluran. Anaethesist 35: 456–472, 1986
5. Kikura M, Ikeda T, Kazama T, Ikeda K. Effect of prostaglandin E_1 on myocardial contractility in dogs anesthetized with halothane: Load independent and noninvasive assessment using transesophageal echocardiography. J Cardiothorac Vasc Anesth 6: 586–592, 1992
6. Kikura M, Ikeda K. Comparison of effects of sevoflurane-nitrous oxide and enflurane-nitrous oxide on myocardial contractility in humans: Load-independent and noninvasive assessment with transesophageal echocardiography. Anesthesiology 79: 235–243, 1993
7. Goertz AW, Seeling W, Heinrich H, Lindner KH, Schmer U. Influence of high thoracic epidural anesthesia on left ventricular contractility assessed using the end-systolic pressure-length relationship. Acta Anesthesiol Scand 37: 38–44, 1993

8. Huemer G, Kolev N, Kurz A, Zimpfer M. Influence of positive end-expiratory pressure on right and left ventricular performance assessed by Doppler two-dimensional echocardiography. Chest 106: 67–73, 1994

9. Kolev N, Usunov G, Vlasakov V. Hemodynamic and pharmacologic influences on the left ventricular echo dimension-pressure loop in dogs. J Cardiography (Tokyo) 14: 537–542, 1984

10. Borow K. Assessment of left ventricular performance. In: Oldershow T, ed. Textbook of adult and pediatric two-dimensional and Doppler echocardiography. Blackwell, London, pp 97–109, 1989

11. Erbel R. Principles of global left ventricular function analysis. In: Roelandt JRT, Sutherland GR, Iliceto S, Linker DT, eds. Cardiac Ultrasound. Churchill Livingstone, Edinburgh, London, pp 219–231, 1993

12. Suter PM, Fairley HB, Isenberg MD. Optimum end-expiratory airway pressure in patients with acute pulmonary failure. N Engl J Med 292: 284–292, 1975

13. Schuster AH, Nanda NC. Doppler echocardiography in cardiac pacing. PACE 5:607–609, 1982

14. Foote GA, Schabel SI, Hodges M. Pulmonary complications of the flow-directed balloon-tipped catheter. N Engl J Med 290: 927–931, 1974

15. Kolev N, Lazarova M, Lengyel M. Doppler determination of right ventricular output and diastolic filling. J Cardiogr (Tokyo) 16: 569–667, 1986

16. Schuster AH, Nanda NC. Doppler evaluation of cardiac output. In: Nanda NC, ed. Doppler echocardiography. 2nd ed, Lea & Febiger, Philadelphia, London, pp 103–106, 1993

17. Vuillle C, Weyman AE. Left ventricle I: General considerations, assessment of chamber size and function. In: Weyman, ed. Principles and practice of echocardiography, 2nd ed. Lea & Febiger, Philadelphia, Baltimore, London, p 605, 1994

18. Kolev N, Huemer G, Steiner W, Leitner K. On-line assessment of left ventricular volumes and ejection fraction by automated boundary detection and backscatter imaging. J Cardiovasc Diag Proc (NY) 11: 141–145, 1993

19. Assmann PE. Quantitative echocardiographic analysis of global and regional left ventricular function: a problem revisited. J Am Soc Echocardiog 3: 478–482, 1990

20. Clements FM, Harpole DH, Quill T, Jones RH, McCann RL. Estimation of left ventricular volume and ejection fraction by two-dimensional echocardiography: Comparison of short axis imaging and simultaneous radionuclide angiography. Br J Anaesth 64: 331–336, 1990

21. Smith MD. Value and limitations of transesophageal echocardiography in determination of left ventricular volumes and ejection fraction. J Am Coll Cardiol 19: 1213–1219, 1992

22. Katz WE, Gasior TA, Quinland JJ, Gorscan III. Transgastric continuous wave Doppler to determine cardiac output. Am J Cardiol 71:853–857, 1993

23. Darmon PL, Hillel Z, Mogtabar A, Mindich B, Thys D. Cardiac output by transesophageal echocardiography using continuous wave Doppler across the aortic valve. Anesthesiology 80: 796–805, 1994

24. Gorcsan J II, Diana P, Ball BA, Hattler BG. Intraoperative determination of cardiac output by transesophageal continuous wave Doppler. Am Heart J 123: 171–176, 1992

25. Muhiudeen IA, Kuecherer HF, Lee E, Cahalan MK, Schieller NB. Intraoperative estimation of cardiac output by transesophageal pulsed Doppler echocardiography. Anesthesiology 79: 9–14, 1991

25a. Akamatsu S, Kondo Y, Ueda N, Takeda N, Takeda T, Dohi S. Continuos cardiac output measurements with newly developed pulmonary artery Doppler catheter (Abstr). Anesthesiology 81(Suppl): A515, 1994

26. Kolev N, Zimpfer M. Impact of ischemia on diastolic function: Clinical relevance and recent Doppler echocardiographic results. Eur J Anaesth (in press), 1995

27. Castor G, Klocke K, Stoll M, Helms J, Niedermark I. Simultaneous measurements of cardiac output by thermodilution, thoracic electrical impedance and Doppler ultrasound. Br J Anaesth 72: 133–138, 1994

28. Fisher DC, Sahn DJ, Friedman MJ. The effect of variations on pulsed Doppler sampling site on calculations of cardiac output. An experimental study in open-chest dogs. Circulation 67: 370–379, 1983

29. Schuster S, Erbel R, Weilemann LS, Lu W, Wellek S. Monitoring during PEEP ventilation in patients with severe left ventricular failure using transesophageal echocardiography. In: Erbel R, ed. Transesophageal echocardiography. Springer, Berlin, Heidelberg, pp 206–217, 1989

30. Kumar A, Minagoe S, Thangathurai D. Noninvasive measurement of cardiac output during surgery using a new continuous wave Doppler esophageal probe. Am J Cardiol 64: 793–782, 1989

31. Haude M, Gerber T, Brennecke R, Erbel R, Meyer J. Continuous and noninvasive monitoring of cardiac output by transesophageal Doppler ultrasound. In: Erbel R, ed. Transesophageal echocardiography. Springer, Berlin, Heidelberg, pp 260–2266, 1989

32. Kumar A, Minagoe, S, Thangathurai D, Mikhali M, Novia D, Vilijoen JF, Rachimtoola SH, Chandraratna PAN. Noninvasive measurement of cardiac output during surgery using a new continuous wave Doppler esophageal probe. Am J Cardiol 64: 739–798, 1989

33. Hoit BD, Rashwan M, Watt C, Sahn D, Bharvgrara V. Calculating cardiac output from transmitral volume flow using Doppler and M-mode echocardiography. Am J Cardiol 62: 131–135, 1988

34. Smith JS, Cahalan MK, Benefield DJ, Byrd BF, Lurz FW, Shapiro WA, Roizen MF, Bouchard MF, Schieller NB. Intraoperative detection of myocardial ischemia in high risk patients. Electrocardiography versus two-dimensional transesophageal echocardiography. Circulation 72: 1015–1021, 1985

35. Robotham JL, Takata M, Berman M, Harasawa Y. Ejection fraction revisited. Anesthesiology 74: 172–183, 1991

36. de Bruijn NP, Clements FM, Kisslo JA. Intraoperative transesophageal color flow mapping: Initial experience. Anesth Analg 66: 386–390, 1987

37. Mangano DT. Preoperative assessment. In: Kaplan JA, ed. Cardiac Anesthesia. 2nd ed. WB Saunders, Philadelphia, pp 341–392, 1987

38. Baron JF, Coriat P, Mundler TM, Bousseau D, Viars P. Left ventricular global and regional function during lumbar epidural anesthesia in patients with and without angina pectoris. Influence of volume loading. Anesthesiology 66: 621–627, 1987

39. Thys DM, Kaplan JA. Cardiovascular physiology. In: Miller RD, ed. Anesthesia. 3rd ed. Churchill Livingstone, New York, pp 551–583, 1990

40. Grein C, Roewer N, Laux G, Schulte J. Perioperative assessment of myocardial contractility by transesophageal echocardiography (Abstr). Anesthesiology 79: A547, 1993

41. Connelly GP, Arkoff H, Dempsey A, Gillespie D. Left ventricular diastolic dysfunction associated with infrarenal aortic crossclamp (Abstr). Anesthesiology 79: A86, 1993

42. Fontes ML, Leung J, Mangano DT, SPI Study Group. Should transesophageal echocardiography monitoring be used routinely in the cardiac intensive care unit (Abstr)? Anesthesiology 79: A288, 1993

43. Ryan T, Burwash I, Graham M, Otto C, Hofer B, Verier E, Spiess B. Is agreement of transesophageal echocardiographic fractional area change and radionuclide ejection fraction dependent on ventricular function (Abstr). Anesthesiology 79: A67, 1993

44. Berguist BD, Lemon KW, Bellows WH, Leung JM, SPI Study Group. Real-time determination of ejection fraction by transesophageal echocardiography: How accurate are 'eyeball' estimates (Abstr)? Anesthesiology 79: A69, 1993

45. Stamm RB, Carabello BA, Mayers DL, Martin NP. Two-dimensional echocardiographic measurement of left ventricular ejection fraction: prospective analysis of what constitutes an adequate determination . Am Heart J 104–109, 1982

46. Erbel R, Krebs W, Henn G, Schweizer P, Richter HA, Meyer J, Effert S. Comparison of single-plane and biplane volume determination by two-dimensional echocardiography. Eur Heart J 3: 469–574, 1982

47. Amoore JH, Santamore WP. Model studies of the contribution of ventricular interdependence of the transient changes in ventricular function with respiratory effort. Cardiovasc Res 23: 683–687, 1989

48. Antani JA, Wayne HH, Kuzman WJ. Ejection phase indexes by invasive and noninvasive methods: an apexcardiographic, echocardiographic and ventriculographic study. Am J Cardiol 43: 239–243, 1979

49. Kolev N. Evaluation of contractile state of the left ventricle from the peak of the first derivative of the apex cardiogram. Am Heart J 100: 600–604, 1980

50. Chen C, Rodriguez L, Cuerrero L, Marshall S, Levine RA, Weyman AE, Thomas JD. Noninvasive estimation of instantaneous first derivative of left ventricular pressure using continuous wave Doppler echocardiography. Circulation 83: 2101–2110, 1991

51. Bove AA, Santamore WP. Mechanical performance of the heart: In: Giulian ER, Fuster V, Gersh BJ, McCoon MD, McCoon DC, eds. Cardiology. Fundamental and practice, 2nd ed. Mosby, St Louis, Baltimore, 1987, pp 154–157.

52. Kolev N, Zimpfer M, Black AM. Ventricular function curves revisited. Eur J Anaesth (in press), 1995

53. Shuga H, Sagawa K. Determinants of instantaneous pressure in canine left ventricle: time and volume specification. Circul Res 46: 256–259, 1980

54. Huemer G, Kolev N, Zimpfer M. Echocardiographic assessment of left ventricular systolic function – the anesthesiologist's view. Eur J Anaesth 11: 437–441, 1994

55. Goertz AW, Lindner KH, Seefelder C, Schirmer U, Beyer M, Georgieff M. Effect of phenylephrine bolus administration on global left ventricular function in patients with coronary artery disease and patients with valvular aortic stenosis. Anesthesiology 78: 834–841, 1993

56. Gorcsan J, Denault A, Gasior TA, Mandarino WA, Kancel MJ, Deneault LG, Hattler BG, Pinsky MR. Rapid estimation of left ventricular contractility from end-systolic relations by echocardiographic automated border detection and femoral arterial pressure. Anesthesiology 81: 553–562, 1994

57. Parker MM, Ognibene FP, Parrillo JE Peak-systolic pressure/end-systolic volume ratio, a load-independent measure of ventricular function, is reversely decreased in human septic shock. Crit Care Med 22: 1955–1959, 1994

58. Carabello BA, Spann JF. The use and limitations of end-systolic indexes of left ventricular function. Circulation 69: 1058–1064, 1984

59. Zimpfer M, Kolev N. Positive inotropic and vasoactive drugs: their therapeutic use in perioperative heart failure. Int J Anaesth (in press) 1994

Chapter 7

Perioperative myocardial ischemia

Cardiac risk

Coronary artery disease (CAD) continues to be one of the most significant diseases confronting the anesthetist. The incidence of CAD in surgical patients is high, and perioperative myocardial ischemia remains the most important cause of cardiac morbidity and mortality, particularly in the increasing subset of older patients who undergo major general surgical procedures. Intra- and postoperative myocardial ischemia has been found to occur in 40–60% of echocardiographically monitored patients with CAD undergoing noncardiac surgery.[1-6] Although the estimated prevalence of cardiovascular disease in Western industrialized countries is approximately 25%, patients requiring surgical procedures are more likely to have cardiovascular disease than the average person.[7] It has been established that approximately 25% of all noncardiac surgical patients require major intraabdominal, thoracic, vascular, neurosurgical or orthopedic procedures, and underlying cardiac conditions (coronary artery disease) may be even more common in this group. Therefore, perioperative cardiac assessment and perioperative cardiac management for patients having noncardiac surgery are common concerns for surgeons and anesthetists.

Clinicians have spent a considerable amount of time stratifying patients with CAD who have surgery into those who may be at higher than average or lower than average risk. Risk stratification has three purposes.[7] The first is to identify patients for whom the cardiac risks are so high that they outweigh the potential benefit of therapy, thus indicating a more conservative surgical approach. The second purpose is to identify patients with clinical problems that may be corrected before surgery. The third purpose is to identify those who are most likely to benefit from risk-reducing interventions such as extensive hemodynamic monitoring.

Historically, risk indices for quantifying perioperative predictors have been reported by the American Society of Anesthesiologists (ASA)[8] (Table 7.1), the New York Heart Association (NYHA),[9] and the Canadian Cardiovascular Society[10] (Table 7.1). In 1977, Goldman et al.[11] released a landmark study in which the authors evaluated 1,001 patients preoperatively and followed their postoperative cardiac outcome. They identified nine preoperative variables that independently predicted cardiac outcome and assigned them a relative predictive value. The variables and their point values are shown in Table 7.2. They placed patients in four cardiac risk index (CRI) categories based on their total perioperative variable score (Table 7.3).

Table 7.1. Classification of coronary artery disease

Class	New York Heart Association	Canadian Cardiovascular Society
I	Patients with cardiac disease but without resulting limitations of physical activity. Ordinary physical activity does not cause undue fatigue, palpitation, angina pain.	Ordinary physical activity, such as walking and climbining stairs, does not cause angina. Angina with rapid exertion at work or recreation.
II	Patients with cardiac disease resulting in slight limitation of physical activity. They are comfortable at rest. Ordinary physical activity results in fatigue, palpitations, angina or dyspnea.	Slight limitation of ordinary activity. Angina caused by walking or climbing stairs rapidly, walking uphill, in cold. Also caused by walking more than two blocks on level ground and climbing more than one flight.
III	Patients with cardiac disease resulting in marked limitation of activity. They are comfortable at rest. Less than ordinary physical activity causes fatigue, palpitations, dyspnea or anginal pain.	Marked limitation of ordinary physical activity. Angina caused by walking one or two blocks on level ground and climbing one flight in normal conditions.
IV	Patients with cardiac disease resulting in inability to carry on physical activity without discomfort. Symptoms of cardiac insufficiency or of anginal syndrome may be present even at rest. If any physical activity is undertaken, discomfort is increased.	Inability to carry on any physical activity without discomfort. Anginal syndrome may be present at rest.

Sources: American Society of Anesthesiologists,[8] the New York Heart Association (NYHA),[9] and the Canadian Cardiovascular Society.[10]

The CRI provides significant predictive potential. Since Goldman's landmark study several investigators have evaluated the validity of the indices, widening the overview in this field with a large number of prospective and retrospective studies. Recently, Roizen[12] and Mangano[13] have reviewed this subject, and they have described the most accurate predictive factors for perioperative cardiac mortality (Table 7.4). While the results of these and other studies are still somewhat controversial, generally, a history of recent myocardial infarction, patterns of unstable angina, ECG left-axis deviation with ST-T wave changes at rest, cardiomegaly on x-ray, and congestive heart failure are believed to affect perioperative outcome. The lack of consistent clinical-pathologic correlation in CAD makes the use of clinical signs listed in Tables 7.1 to 7.4 difficult for definitively assessing perioperative prognosis. Therefore, the identification of reliable predictors is essential to make a definitive estimation of risk. Stress ECG testing, with its low cost and ease of performance, is still considered very effective.

Dipyridamole thallium[14] has been legitimized as a valid predictive test for patients in the intermediate-risk categories. High sensitivity was attributed to the test when it was used to predict morbidity in patients undergoing vascular surgery. More recently, other investigators[15] demonstrated a low sensitivity of dipyridamole thallium testing. Therefore, some authors[16] do not regard this test as predictive.

Table 7.2. Goldman's computation of cardiac risk index

Variable	Point value
History	
Age > 70 yr	5
MI in previous 6 mo	10
Physical examination	
S_3 gallop or JVD	11
Aortic stenosis	3
Electrocardiogram	
Rhythm other than sinus or PACs on last ECG	7
> 5 PVCs/min documented at any time before operation	7
General status	
$PO_2 < 60$ or $PCO_2 > 50$ mmHg	
$K^+ < 3.0$ or $HCO_3 < 20$ mEq/l	
BUN > 50 or Cr > 3.0 mg/100 ml	
Abnormal SGOT, signs of chronic liver disease	3
Operation	
Intraperitoneal, intrathoracic, or aortic	3
Emergency	4
Total possible	53

JVD jugular venous distention; *PAC* premature atrial contractions; *PO$_2$* oxygen tension; *HCO$_3$* bicarbonate; *BUN* blood urea nitrogen; *Cr* creatinine; *SGOT* serum glutamic oxaloacetic transaminase; *MI* myocardial infaction; *PAC* premature atrial contraction; PVC premature ventricular contraction
Source: Goldman et al.[11]

Table 7.3 Cardiac risk index (CRI)

CRI class	Total predictive points	Risk of cardiac death (%)
I	0–5	0.2
II	6–12	2.0
III	13–25	2.0
IV	≥ 26	56

Source: Goldman et al.[11]

A review of the Coronary Artery Surgery Study (CASS)[10] registry data in patients who subsequently underwent noncardiac surgery reveals that the presence of poor ventricular function (angiographic cardiac output, ejection fraction and Frank-Starling function curves) was the only independent predictor of perioperative risk.

Table 7.4. Perioperative cardiac morbidity: historical predictors

Roizen[12]	Mangano[13]
Age	Age (controversial)
Angina (NYHA and CCS evaluation); ST, T, QRS abnormalities	Angina (controversial)
Recent MI (within 6 months)	Previous MI
Congestive heart failure, cardiomegaly	Congestive heart failure
Heart rhythm other than sinus, PACs, PVCs > 5/min	Dysrhythmia Rhythm other than sinus
Aortic stenosis, Mitral regurgitation	Valvular heart disease
BUN > 50 mg/100 ml, K$^+$ < 3.0 mEq/l	Hypertension (controversial) Diabetes mellitus Peripheral vascular disease

NYHA New York Heart Association; *CCS* Canadian Cardiovascular Society.
Sources: Roizen[12] and Mangano.[13]

Coronary anatomy was not an independent predictor of outcome. Now that ventricular function data can be obtained using echocardiography, it is time to widen the risk criteria by employing two-dimensional Doppler echocardiography.

References

1. Massie BM, Mangano DT. Assessment of perioperative risk: Have we put the cart before the horse? J Am Coll Cardiol 21: 1353–1356, 1993
2. Hollenberg M, Mangano DT, Browner WS, London MJ, Tubau JF, Tateo IM. Predictors of postoperative myocardial ischemia in patients undergoing noncardiac surgery. JAMA 268: 205–209, 1992
3. Raby KE, Barry J, Creager MA, Cook F, Weisberg MC, Goldman L. Detection and significance of intraoperative and postoperative myocardial ischemia in peripheral vascular surgery. JAMA 268: 222–227, 1992
4. Abraham SA, Coles A, Coley CM, Strauss HW, Boucher CA, Eagle K. Coronary risk of noncardiac surgery. Progr Cardiovasc Dis 34: 205–234, 1991
5. Mangano DT, Browner WS, Holloenberg MH, London MJ, Tubau JF, Tateo IM. Association of perioperative myocardial ischemia with cardiac morbidity and mortality in men undergoing noncardiac surgery. N Engl J Med 323: 1781–1788, 1990
6. Ouyang P, Gerstenblith G, Furman WR, Gloueke PJ, Gottlieb SO. Frequency and significance of early postoperative silent myocardial ischemia in patients having peripheral vascular surgery. Am J Cardiol 64: 1113–1116, 1989
7. Wong T, Detsky AS. Perioperative cardiac risk assessment for patients having peripheral vascular surgery. Ann Int Med 116: 743–753, 1992

8. American Society of Anesthesiologists. New classification of physical status. Anesthesiology24: 111–119, 1963
9. Criteria Committee of the NYHA. Diseases of the Heart and Blood Vessels: Nomenclature and Criteria for Diagnosis. 6th ed. Little, Brown, Boston, 1964
10. Coronary Artery Surgery Study (CASS). Manual of Operations II: Data collecting and storage. Collaborative studies in coronary artery surgery. Washington, DC: National Heart, Lung, Institute. Prepared by the CASS Coordinating Center, 1978
11. Goldman L, Caldera DL, Nussbaum SR. Multifactoral index of cardiac risk in noncardiac surgical procedures. N Engl J Med 297: 845–848, 1977
12. Roizen MF. Anesthetic implications of concurrent diseases. In: Miller RD, ed. Anesthesia. 3rd ed. Churchill Livingstone, New York, pp 793–893, 1990
13. Mangano DT. Perioperative cardiac morbidity. Anesthesiology 72: 153–157, 1990
14. Boucher CA, Brewser DC, Darling C, Okada RD, Strauss HW, Pohost GM. Determination of cardiac risk by dipyridamole thallium imaging before peripheral vascular surgery. N Engl J Med 312: 389–392, 1985
15. McEnroe CS, O'Donnel TF Jr, Yeager A. Comparison of ejection fraction and Goldman risk factors analysis to dipyridamole-thallium 201 studies in the evaluation of cardiac morbidity after aortic aneurysm surgery. J Vasc Surg 11: 497–502, 1990
16. Coriat P. Dipyridamole-thallium imaging—no routine test prior to vascular surgery. Society of Cardiovascular Anesthesiologists, 13th Annual Meeting, 1991

Myocardial ischemia: pathophysiology and effects of the inhalational anesthetics

The major complications of noncardiac surgery-death, myocardial infarction, transient myocardial ischemia, congestive heart failure and unstable angina pectoris are in most cases directly or indirectly related to underlying coronary artery disease. Several factors are responsible for perioperative ischemia. These include marked hemodynamic fluctuations, fluid shifts, hypercoagulable state, hypoxemia, catecholamine changes, altered vasomotor regulation and activation of other neurohormonal pathways.[1-6] It is unclear whether the anesthetic *per se* prevents or causes these physiologic changes and complications. The currently available inhalational anesthetics agents include halothane, enflurane, isoflurane, and nitrous oxide. Additionally, two new inhalational agents, desflurane and sevoflurane, are in the final stages of clinical trials and may soon be introduced into clinical practice.

Nitrous oxide (N_2O) effects on the coronary circulation and myocardial ischemia are controversial. Several studies in animal experiments demonstrated that N_2O may have deleterious effects on myocardial oxygen supply.[7,8] Other human studies, however, have shown minimal or no effect of N_2O on myocardial ischemia. Cahalan- et al.[9] demonstrated no detectable changes in regional wall motion abnormalities by TEE and ECG. Preexisting poor myocardial function also does not seem to predispose to N_2O-induced ischemia.[10]

All of the **volatile inhalational anesthetics** decrease myocardial oxygen demand (MVO_2). Halothane and enflurane decrease MVO_2 more than does isoflurane.[11] However, when halothane was added to N_2O in a heart with a critical coronary stenosis, it caused worsening of regional myocardial dysfunction.[12] In addition to a decrease in MVO_2, isoflurane may cause a maldistribution of coronary blood flow and worsen ischemia[13] (see below). Isoflurane has been shown to improve tolerance to pacing-induced myocardial ischemia in humans,[14] presumably by decreasing MVO_2, although other recent studies have shown only halothane and enflurane to decrease MVO_2, while isoflurane had no effect.[15] Furthermore, in a dog model, halothane but not isoflurane offered protection from total myocardial ischemia. Recently, it has been shown that desflurane and sevoflurane[16] both decrease MVO_2, in a manner similar to that of isoflurane.

Isoflurane is a potent coronary vasodilator and will increase coronary blood flow out of proportion to the increase in MVO_2. This is in contrast to halothane, which will increase coronary blood flow in response to an increase in MVO_2.[17] Desflurane caused an increase in coronary blood flow, though not as much as isoflurane.[18] On the other hand, Merin et al.[19] showed the increase in coronary blood flow to be similar for desflurane and isoflurane. While sevoflurane is also a coronary vasodilator and will increase coronary blood flow, some authors suggest that its effect may not be as pronounced as that of isoflurane.[16] Other studies have shown sevoflurane's effect on coronary blood flow to be very similar to that of isoflurane.[20]

Whether or not isoflurane causes coronary steal has been the subject of much controversy in the anesthetic literature. Giving the fact that isoflurane is the small vessel type coronary vasodilator, it should come as no surprise that it is capable of producing myocardial ischemia. Although seemingly paradoxical, it is well known that this type of coronary vasodilator can cause myocardial ischemia by delivering flow away from areas of borderline perfusion and limited coronary reserve toward areas that are already adequately perfused. This phenomenon has been termed (*inter*)coronary or *transmural* "steal"[21,22] and has been convincingly demonstrated to occur in a variety of animal models.[23,24] Pharmacologically, isoflurane belongs to the class of vasodilators having predominantly small coronary (*resistance*) vessel effects, with little or no action on large epicardial (*conductance*) vessels. Other compounds in this class include adenosine, dipyramidole, papaverine and carbo- chromen.[23] In contrast, effective antiischemic agents, such as nitrates and calcium channel blocking agents, have predominant effects on the large epicardial arteries.[24]

What is a coronary steal phenomenon? Pathophysiologically, the coronary steal phenomenon is a nonspecific mechanism. It has been observed that when coronary perfusion pressure (aortic diastolic pressure minus left ventricular end-diastolic pressure) falls below the critical levels of 60 to 70 mm Hg, the coronary vessels become maximally dilated and flow becomes pressure-dependent, i.e., autoregulation is lost.[21] This observation underlines the importance of maintaining coronary perfusion pressure in patients with hypotension or vasodilation in any case, but especially in those with regional wall motion abnormalities. The mechanism responsible for vasodilation-induced ischemia is likely to be flow reduction in the region supplied by the stenotic coronary artery. Four main mechanisms possibly resulting in a decrease in myocardial oxygen supply have been suggested:

— transmural steal or vertical steal;
— intercoronary (myocardial) steal or horizontal steal;
— systemic steal;
— luxury perfusion.

Transmural steal or vertical steal. One of the interesting aspects of atherosclerotic lesions is that even in the presence of a fixed anatomical stenosis, resistance is not fixed.[25,26] Because myocardial oxygen demands of the endocardium are greater than those of the epicardium, the resistance vessels of the endocardium are more dilated than those of the epicardium. A vasodilator stimulus may then decrease resistance in the subepicardial but not in subendocardial vessels because the subendocardial vasodilator reserve is already exhausted.[26] Even if total blood flow increases, the net effect is shunting of blood from the subendocardium to the subepicardium, ultimately resulting in myocardial ischemia. This explanation has been substantiated by clinical evidence.[27] Patients with single-vessel disease of the left anterior descending artery exhibited the mechanical manifestation of myocardial ischemia (regional systolic wall motion abnormalities) associated with an increase in anterior coronary flow, although to a much lesser extent than in patients with normal coronary arteries or patients with coronary disease and a negative dipyridamole-echocardiography test.

Intercoronary (myocardial) steal or horizontal steal. In the presence of coronary occlusion, it seems conceivable that arteriolar vasodilators might have no effect: "Opening the taps wider (i.e., peripheral vasodilation) will not alter the rate at which the bath fills if the water is turned off at a main.''[28] Unfortunately, the hydraulics of the coronary tree are more complex for several reasons, such as the presence of collateral circulation. When vasodilators act mainly on the small (*resistance*) coronary vessels, they can fully dilate the resistance vessels of the unoccluded artery and thereby increase the pressure gradient along the vessel. In the situation (Fig. 7.1) in which a partial stenosis of the vessel feeding the collaterals (distal from total stenosis) exists, the small pressure drop across the stenosis present under baseline conditions increases, and thereby the pressure at the point of origin of the collateral vessels decreases. Such a reduction in collateral perfusion pressure decreases collateral blood flow to the myocardium dependent upon the occluded artery.[26]

Systemic steal. In the presence of severe coronary artery disease and decreased diastolic perfusion pressure, the lowering of arteriolar peripheral resistance (nitroprusside > nifidepine > isoflurane/sevoflurane > enflurane/halothane) can lead to a coronary steal diverting perfusion from an ischemic coronary vascular bed to a preferentially dilated peripheral vascular bed.[28]

Luxury perfusion. After vasodilation, a paradoxical situation takes place. The flow is regionally augmented, but cannot be used by the metabolism of the myocardial cell, which then suffers oxygen "hunger amidst affluence." This can result from the preferential opening of nonnutritional pathways in the microcirculation.[2]

Getting back to the volatile inhalation anesthetics, in spite of reports from some authors[29,30] that isoflurane can cause coronary steal, several recent studies have shown no effect on coronary steal by isoflurane.[31-33] There is even some evidence that isoflurane may be protective for the ischemic heart. As discussed earlier, Tarnow et al.[14] showed that isoflurane protects against pacing-induced myocardial ischemia. Other investigators demonstrated that isoflurane decreased the area of myocardial necrosis[34] or improved recovery of a stunned myocardium in the dog model.[35]

Whatever the mechanism for intra- and postoperative myocardial ischemia is, it is now clear that CAD provides only the substrate for each of these mechanisms.[1] The

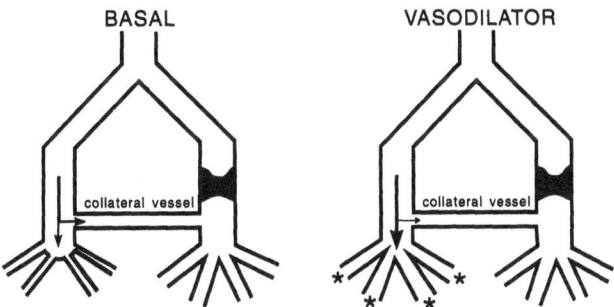

Fig. 7.1. Schematic representation of a mechanism of intercoronary (horizontal) steal. The dilation of the vascular bed distally after moderate stenosis (*) causes shunting of blood through these vessels (thick arrow) at the expense of the collateral myocardial circulation (thin arrow)

underlying pathology actually differs among patients with CAD. Thus, ischemia owing to an increase in metabolic demand is most likely to occur in patients with preexisting critical coronary stenosis or occluded coronary arteries with myocardium supplied by collateral vessels. Ischemia due to decreased oxygen supply may occur in these patients, but it also may occur in patients with less critical stenosis, because it is very likely that thrombotic occlusions occur more frequently in vessels that were previously not severely obstructed, as in the case of myocardial infarction in nonsurgical patients.[36] Patients with prior myocardial infarction, though they may not be vulnerable to further ischemia, are certainly in jeopardy for developing heart failure and pulmonary edema.[2] Thus, the presence of coronary disease, but not necessarily preexisting critical stenosis, is the substrate for most perioperative cardiac events.

References

1. Massie BM, Mangano DT. Assessment of perioperative risk: Have we put the cart before the horse? J Am Coll Cardiol 21: 1353–1356, 1993
2. Hollenberg M, Mangano DT, Browner WS, London MJ, Tubau JF, Tateo IM. Predictors of postoperative myocardial ischemia in patients undergoing noncardiac surgery. JAMA 268: 205–209, 1992
3. Raby KE, Barry J, Creager MA, Cook F, Weisberg MC, Goldman L. Detection and significance of intraoperative and postoperative myocardial ischemia in peripheral vascular surgery. JAMA 268: 222–227, 1992
4. Abraham SA, Coles A, Coley CM, Strauss HW, Boucher CA, Eagle K. Coronary risk of noncardiac surgery. Progr Cardiovasc Dis 34: 205–234, 1991
5. Ouyang P, Garstenblith G, Furman WR, Gloueke PJ, Gottlieb SO. Frequency and significance of early postoperative silent myocardial ischemia in patients having vascular surgery. Am J Cardiol 64: 1113–1116, 1989
6. Mangano DT, Browner WS, Hollenberg MH, London MJ, Tubau JF, Tateo IM. Association of perioperative myocardial ischemia with cardiac morbidity and mortality in men undergoing noncardiac surgery. N Engl J Med 323: 1781–1788, 1990
7. Cason BA, Demas KA, Mazer CD. Effects of nitrous oxide on coronary pressure and regional contractile function in experimental myocardial ischemia. Anesth Analg 72: 604–611, 1991
8. Nathan HJ. Nitrous oxide worsens myocardial ischemia in isoflurane-anesthetized dogs. Anesthesiology 68: 707–715, 1988
9. Cahalan MC, Prakash O, Rulf ENR. Addition of nitous oxide to fentanyl anesthesia does not induce myocardial ischemia in patients with ischemic heart disease. Anesthesiology 67: 925–927, 1987
10. Mitchell MM, Prakash O, Rulf ENR. Nitrous oxide does not induce myocardial ischemia in patients with ischemic heart disease and poor ventricular function. Anesthesiology 71: 526–534, 1989
11. Bosnjak ZJ, Aggarwal A, Turner LA. Differential effects of halothane, enflurane and isoflurane on Ca^{++} transients and papillary muscle tension in guinea pigs. Anesthesiology 76: 123–131, 1992
12. Leone BJ, Philbin DM, Lehhot JJ. Gradual or abrupt nitrous oxide administration in a canine model of critical coronary stenosis induces regional myocardial dysfunction that is worsened by halothane. Anesth Analg 67: 814–822, 1988
13. Tatekawa S, Traber KB, Hantler CB. Effects of isoflurane on myocardial blood flow, function and oxygen consumption in the presence of critical coronary stenosis in dogs. Anesth Analg 66: 1073–1082, 1987

14. Tarnow J, Markschies-Hornung A, Schulte-Sasse U. Isoflurane improves the tolerance to pacing-induced myocardial ischemia. Anesthesiology 64: 147–156, 1986
15. Stowe DF, Marijic J, Bosnjiak ZJ. Direct comparative effects of halothane, enflurane and isoflurane on oxygen supply and demand in isolated hearts. Anesthesiology 74: 1087–1095, 1991
16. Conzen PF, Vollmar B, Habazett I. Systemic and regional hemodynamic effects of isoflurane and sevoflurane in rats. Anesth Analg 74: 79–88, 1992
17. Kenny D, Proctor LT, Schmeling WT, Kampine JP, Warltier DC. Isoflurane causes only minimal increases in coronary blood flow independent of oxygen demand. Anesthesiology 75: 640–649, 1991
18. Boban M, Stowe DF, Buljubasic N. Direct comparative effects of isoflurane and desflurane in isolated guinea pig hearts. Anesthesiology 76: 775–789, 1992
19. Merin RG, Bernard JM, Doursout MF. Comparison of the effects of isoflurane and desflurane on cardiovascular dynamics and regional blood flow in the chronically instrumented dog. Anesthesiology 74: 568–574, 1991
20. Bernard JM, Wouters PF, Doursout MF. Effects of sevoflurane on cardiac and coronary dynamics in chronically instrumented dogs. Anesthesiology 72: 659–662, 1990
21. Braunwald E, Sobel BE. Coronary blood flow and myocardial ischemia. In: Braunwald E, ed. Heart disease. 4th ed. WB Saunders, Philadelphia, pp 1162–1198, 1992
22. Kolev N, Zimpfer M. Impact of myocardial ischemia on diastolic function. Clinical relevance and recent Doppler echocardiographic results. Eur J Anaesth (in press), 1994
23. Priebe HJ. Isoflurane causes more severe regional myocardial dysfunction than halothane in dogs with a critical coronary artery stenosis. Anesthesiology 69: 72–83, 1988
24. Cohen MV. Coronary steal in awake dogs: a real phenomenon. Cardiovasc Res 16: 339–349, 1982
25. Epstein SE, Cannon RO, Talbot TL. Hemodynamic principles in the control of coronary blood flow (Abstr). Am J Cardiol 56: 4E, 1985
26. Brown BG, Bolson EL, Dodge HT. Dynamic mechanism in human coronary stenosis. Circulation 70: 917–922, 1984
27. Picano E, Simonetti I, Massini M. Transient myocardial dysfunction during pharmacologic vasodilation as an index of reduced coronary reserve: A coronary hemodynamic and echocardiographic study. Am J Coll Cardiol 8: 84–89, 1986
28. Picano E, Lattanzi F, Masisni M, Distante A. Dipyridamole-echocardiography: An alternative form of stress testing for coronary artery disease. In: Kerber RE, ed. Echocardiography in coronary artery disease. Futura, Mount Kisko, p 144, 1988
29. Khambatta HJ, Sonntag H, Larsen R. Global and regional blood flow and metabolism during equipotent halothane and isoflurane anesthesia in patients with coronary artery disease. Anesth Analg 67: 936–942, 1988
30. Diana P, Tullock WC, Gorcsan J, Ferson PF, Arvan S. Myocardial ischemia: A comparison between isoflurane and enflurane in coronary artery bypass patients. Anesth Analg 77: 221–226, 1993
31. Inoue K, Reichelt W, El-Banayosy A, Minami K, Dallman G, Hartmann N, Windeler J. Does isoflurane lead to a higher incidence of myocardial infarction and perioperative death than enflurane in coronary artery surgery? A clinical study of 1178 patients. Anesth Analg 71: 469–474, 1990
32. Leung JM, Coehner P, O'Kelly BF. Isoflurane anesthesia and myocardial ischemia: Comparative risk versus sufentanil anesthesia in patients undergoing coronary artery bypass graft surgery. Anesthesiology 74:938-947, 1991
33. Slogoff S, Keats AS, Dear WE. Steal-prone coronary anatomy and myocardial ischemia associated with four primary anesthetics in humans. Anesth Analg 72: 22–27, 1991
34. Davis RF, Sidi A. Effect of isoflurane on the extent of myocardial necrosis and on systemic hemodynamics, regional metabolism in dogs after coronary artery occlusion. Anesth Analg 69: 575–586, 1989

35. Warltier DC, Al-Wathiqui MH, Kampine JP. Recovery of contractile function of stunned myocardium in chronically instrumented dogs is enhanced by halothane or isoflurane. Anesthesiology 69: 552–565, 1988
36. Little WC, Constantinescu M, Applegate RJ, Kutcher MA, Barrows MT, Kahl FR, Santamore WP. Can coronary angiography predict the site of a subsequent myocardial infarction in patients with mild-to-moderate coronary artery disease? Circulation 78: 1157–1166, 1988

Left ventricular segmental wall motion analysis

Experimental and clinical studies

Tennant and Wiggers[1] first described the association of segmental wall motion abnormalities (SWMA) and myocardial ischemia in 1935. Within seconds after the interruption of myocardial perfusion, normal inward motion and thickening of the affected myocardial wall ceases. Tennant and Wiggers described how ligation of a coronary artery resulted in an almost immediate failure of contraction in the affected area of the myocardium, which progressed to paradoxical wall motion. Many subsequent angiographic studies in animals further refined this observation. For instance, Forrester el al.[2] demonstrated that in the presence of a severe coronary constriction, segmental contraction decreased linearly as a function of segmental coronary blood flow: hypokinesis progressed to dyskinesis as coronary perfusion pressure decreased from 100 to 20 mmHg. The same work group, in another study,[3] found that although hypokinesia appeared first at approximately a 50% reduction in coronary blood flow, ECG changes did not occur until coronary blood flow was reduced by 75%. Comparison of contractile function and ECG changes in the epicardium and endocardium further reveals that contraction abnormalities appear first in the endocardium, preceding the S-T changes from endocardial leads.[4] It is not surprising that ischemic manifestations appear initially in the endocardium. The subendocardium is known to be at greatest risk with coronary artery stenosis.

Battler et al.[5] compared segmental myocardial contraction and S-T segment changes (intracardiac and body surface leads) during ischemia. During mild, partial occlusion of a coronary artery, segmental myocardial contraction decreased in 17% and intracardiac derived S-T segments elevated significantly, but no changes in the body surface ECG occurred for the first 10–12 minutes of partial occlusion. With more severe coronary constriction, systolic wall thickening further decreased and both intracardiac and surface ECGs showed significant S-T changes. However, S-T changes appeared 1 to 5 min after decreases in segmental wall thickening. Until recently, anesthesiologists could not detect these changes because they had no way of directly monitoring myocardial contraction.

The advent of coronary angioplasty has afforded clinical investigators the opportunity to study the time sequence of acute ischemia. The earliest association with coronary flow deprivation is the onset of two-dimensional echocardiographic regional wall motion abnormalities. Hauser et al.[6] studied the sequence of TEE and ECG (seven ECG leads, augmented leads and V_5) changes. The interruption of coronary blood flow by inflation of the dilating balloon produced new SWMA in the distribution of the instrumented coronary artery in 86% of the dilatations. The onset of the wall motion abnormality began approximately 19 sec after coronary occlusion and began to normalize 17 sec after reperfusion. S-T segment changes (seven ECG leads) occurred in 30% of the dilatations approximately 30 sec after coronary artery occlusion. If a comparison between two-dimensional echocardiography and ECG monitoring merely demonstrates differing latencies on the order of seconds, the issue might be considered trivial. However, in a separate publication that also pertained to findings established during angioplasty, Wohlgelernter et al.[7] also demonstrated a relative ischemia detection sensitivity of two-dimensional TEE, as compared with 3-lead and 12-lead ECG monitoring. These findings also pertain to TEE monitoring. Smith et al.[8] compared surface electrocardiography and two-dimensional echocardiography for detection of myocardial ischemia in 50 anesthetized patients known to have coronary artery disease. Twenty four of the 50 patients (48%) developed new segmental wall motion abnormalities intraoperatively; only six (12%), however, developed S-T changes on ECG. S-T changes were always accompanied by wall motion abnormalities, which developed before or simultaneously with the S-T changes. Of the three patients who developed perioperative myocardial infarction, only one had intraoperative S-T changes whereas all had persistent new wall motion abnormalities.

Similar results comparing ECG and two-dimensional echocardiography have been reported by many other investigators.[9-14] Roizen et al.[13] observed frequent SWMA in patients with aortic occlusion at the supraceliac level. These changes were not always detected by traditional monitoring devices, such as pulmonary artery pressure monitoring. In fact, the pulmonary artery wedge pressure was always within normal range, except for a transient increase in two of twelve patients who were undergoing aortic occlusion at the supraceliac level. In a study in which continuous TEE and 2-lead Holter monitoring were used in patients who were undergoing coronary artery surgery, Leung and associates found interesting correlations with hemodynamics.[10] Six of their 50 patients had uninterpretable S-T segments, while no patient had an uninterpretable echocardiogram. During simultaneous TEE and ECG monitoring, 56 new SWMA occurred, of which 8 (14%) were accompanied by S-T segment changes; and 18 S-T segment changes occurred, of which 8 (44%) were accompanied by new SWMA, 4 (22%) by equilocal SWMA (decrease of one class in segmental motion) and 6 (33%) by no change in segmental wall motion. Hemodynamics were monitored continuously, but rarely did a change of more than 20% in heart rate, systemic blood pressure, or pulmonary artery diastolic pressure accompany the onset of a new SWMA or S-T segment change. Six of the 50 patients had major adverse outcomes and all of these six patients had new SWMA detected after cardiopulmonary bypass that persisted to the conclusion of the surgery. All of the six had new S-T segment changes after bypass, and three other had uninterpretable S-T segments due to bundle branch block or ventricular pacing. No patient without a new SWMA that occurred after cardiopulmonary bypass had a major adverse outcome. In a view of these data, one might reasonably question the propriety of using the ECG as a "gold standard" for ischemia. However, the use of regional wall motion abnormalities as an alternate "gold standard" does have its pitfalls,[16] which will be discussed at the end of this chapter as a nonischemic cause for abnormal wall motion, including methodological problems.

In a study of 95 high-risk patients (with coronary artery disease or with two or more risk factors) who were undergoing noncardiac surgery, London and associates[17] used continuous TEE and continuous 12-lead ECG to characterize the incidence of intraoperative myocardial ischemia. They found a relatively high incidence (33%) of new intraopeartive SWMA in these patients with TEE.

Furthermore, abnormalities of regional systolic function are important signs of acute as well as of chronic ischemia. For this reason, only the new SWMA can be used for diagnosis of transient myocardial ischemia or acute coronary insufficiency. The extent and severity of these abnormalities are powerful predictors of the subsequent clinical course in patients undergoing cardiac and noncardiac surgery.[18–21] It has been shown that in patients surviving the acute phase of myocardial infarction, predischarge two-dimensional scores predict 1–2-year outcome as well.[22,23] Division of the left ventricle into standardized segments, a standard nomenclature for degree of asynergy and other conventions promote a unified approach and allow interstudy comparison to be made.

Two-dimensional echocardigraphy is very suitable for the assessment of segmental wall motion because the entire left ventricle can be seen by a combination of views, and especially because it allows visualization of both endocardium and epicardium. Cineangiography, on the other hand, reveals only endocardial motion. Systolic wall motion abnormalities are quantified echocardiographically by endocardial motion, degree of circumferential shortening, and systolic wall thickening. Endocardial movement, representing left ventricular ejection at a global level, can be used to express a regional or segmental ejection fraction.

Standard TEE monitoring position

As discussed in chapter 2, the resolution and display characteristics of individual points along the endocardial and epicardial surface of the left ventricle vary depending on the position of the targets relative to the direction of propagation of the ultrasonic beam. Targets that are perpendicular to the beam reflects sound directly back to the transducer and are resolved using the axial resolution of the system, which depends on transducer frequency and pulse duration. Resolution in this dimension is accurate to the submilimeter level. Targets that are laterally positioned relative to the scan plane are less highly reflective and depend on the lateral resolution of the system for their definition. Lateral resolution depends on beam width, which in turn varies with position along the beam, output power, and receiver gain.

For the transgastric left ventricular short-axis cross-sectional view, targets positioned posteriorly and anteriorly in the ventricle are recorded using the axial resolution of the imaging system, whereas those oriented medially and laterally are imaged using lateral resolution. For the transgastric left ventricular long-axis view, the relationship is shifted by 90°. From the midesophageal left ventricular long-axis view, virtually all endo- and epicardial targets are imaged with the lateral resolution of the system. Because laterally positioned targets are less clearly recorded, areas of echo dropout frequently occurs along the medial and lateral margins the endocardium and especially epicardium.

The standard TEE monitoring position is the left ventricular short-axis cross-section at the level of the papillary muscle (Figs. 7.2 and 7.3). The left ventricular

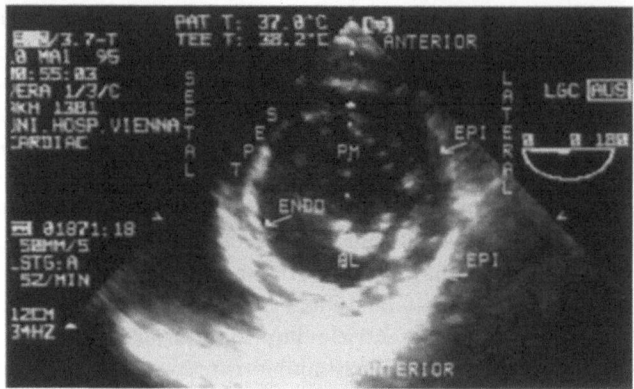

Fig. 7.2. Transgastric left ventricular short-axis view at the level of the papillary muscle during diastole. *PM* posteromedial papillary muscle; *AL* anterolateral papillary muscle; *ENDO* endocardium; *EPI* epicardium; *SEPT* interventricular septum

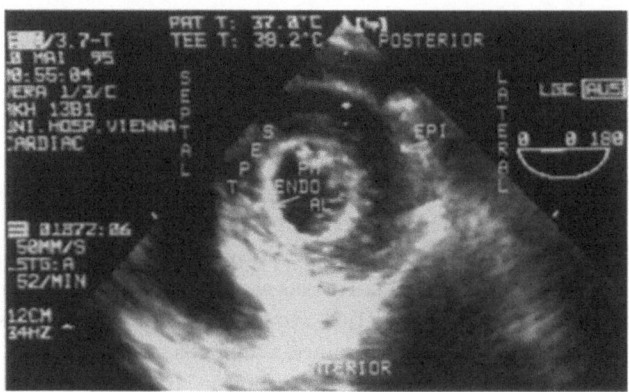

Fig. 7.3. Transgastric left ventricular short-axis view during systole. For abbreviations, see Fig. 7.2

image appears circular in this section, with the interventricular septum accounting for 40% of its circumference.[24] Although the septum constitutes a part of both ventricles, its thickness and spatial configuration suggest that it is an anatomic and functional part of the left ventricle. The echocardiographic image of a short-axis plane in the course of normal contraction shows the pattern briefly described as follows: the single point of endocardium approaches the center of the ventricle; the perimeter bounded by the endocardium and the circular area within the ventricle are reduced in accordance; at the same time the wall thickness increases (Fig. 7.3). Regional wall motion abnormality is a *nonspecific* term applied to a segment of myocardium that demonstrates abnormal contraction or relaxation. The term does not specify the precise nature of the impaired wall motion dynamics, its timing in the cardiac cycle or the technique by which wall motion was studied.

Left ventricular short-axis cross-section is readily obtainable with TEE and it is the best plane for intraoperative and ICU monitoring for four reasons. *First,* all three major coronary arteries supply the myocardium viewed in this cross-section (Fig. 7.4). The septum and the anterior wall are supplied by the left anterior descending (interventricular) artery. The lateral wall (including the anterolateral papillary muscle) is supplied by the circumflex artery. The inferior wall, part of the posterior ventricular septum, and the posteromedial papillary muscle are supplied by the right coronary artery when this is dominant (as in 90% of subjects). When the left coronary artery is dominant, it supplies these latter segments through the terminal branches of the left circumflex artery. *Second,* nine-tenths of stroke volume is derived from shortening in the ventricular short-axis. Very little contribution to the cardiac output results from shortening of the long-axis. *Third,* changes in left ventricular filling cause larger changes in the short-axis dimension than in the long-axis dimension. Thus, changes in filling are more easily appreciated by viewing the short-axis cross-section. *Fourth,* movement of the probe from this position is immediately apparent, because the morphology of the papillary muscles changes as they extend from their origins in the wall of the ventricle to their insertions into the chords.

As yet, there is no generally accepted nomenclature for the myocardial segments as seen in the transesophageal short-axis view. The American Society of Echocardiography has proposed a nomenclature that divides the midpapillary cross-section into octants.[25] Most anesthesiologists, however, have used a division of quadrants[6,9−12]; segments are described as septal, anterior, lateral and inferior

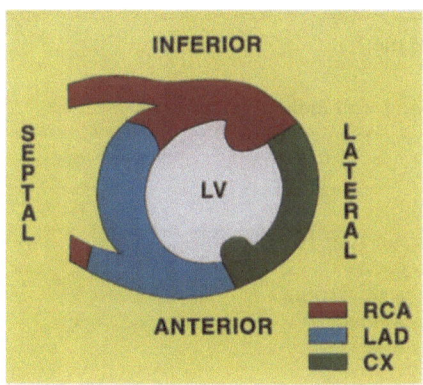

Fig. 7.4. Schematic representation of the left ventricular short-axis cross-section view demonstrating the areas of myocardium that are supplied by the three major coronary arteries. *RCA* right coronary artery; *LAD* left anterior descending (interventricular) artery; *CX* circumflex coronary artery; *LV* left ventricle

(posterior), and the insertion of the right ventricular free wall and the anterolateral papillary muscle are used as anatomical landmarks (Fig. 7.5). Some authors use both papillary muscles as landmarks for a division into quadrants, but it must be remembered that when such a definition is adopted, these are applicable at an angle of approximately 130°, rather than 90°.

A segment is considered suitable for wall motion analysis if 70% of its entire outline is visible continuously throughout systole and diastole. The wall motion of each of the segments is graded quantitatively Table 7.5 after Cahalan[26] and van Daele and Roelandt[27] or semiquantitatively Table 7.6 after Stanley.[28]

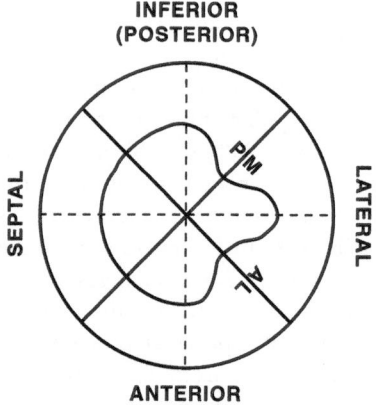

Fig. 7.5. Division of the short-axis view of the left ventricle into four segments or eight subsegments, as recommended by the American Society of Echocardiography. *PM* postero-medial papillary muscle; *AL* anterolateral papillary muscle

Table 7.5. Quantitative segmental wall motion scoring system

	Radial shortening	Myocardial thickening	Scores
Normal motion	>30%	+++	0
Mild hypokinesis	10–30%	++	1
Severe hypokinesis	>0 but <10%	+	2
Akinesis	0	0	3
Dyskinesis	systolic lengthening or bulging out	systolic thinning	4

Sources: Cahalan[26] and van Daele and Roelandt[27].

Table 7.6. Semiquantitative (subjective) segmental wall motion scoring

	Meaning	Scores
Normal	no evidence of dysfunction	0
Mild hypokinesis	minimal diminutions in function	1
Severe hypokinesis	barely perceptible movement	2
Akinesis	total lack of movement or thickening	3
Dyskinesis	paradoxical outward movement or wall thinning	4

Source: Stanley[28].

Although semiquantitative method is attractive because of its simplicity, visual-based approach depends on the skill and experience of the observer and therefore may lack objectivity. Further, this approach does not provide truly quantitative data concerning function within abnormal zones and, hence, does not relate degrees of dysfunction to changes in perfusion. Despite these limitations, the well trained eye is extremely sensitive in separating abnormal from normal function.

Because of need for objective, reproducible, and quantitative means of assessing the extent and severity of abnormal regional function, quantitative approach for measuring the parameters have to be used. Although seemingly simple, this has been proven to be enormously difficult, involving many fundamental choices as well as theoretic and technical problems (see below). Before discussing the various methods for measuring regional function, however, it is important to remember that all of the factors discussed become important because the absolute changes in motion and thickening measured are very small (in the range of 1 to 5 mm). Because function is generally expressed as a percentage of end-diastolic value for the chosen parameter, the degree of magnification is determined by the denominator of the fractional expression. Because of these small numbers and the large relative errors they produce, it is important that all the potential sources of error be considered and eliminate for these measurement to be meaningful as possible.

An echo episode suggestive of ischemia is defined when wall motion of any segment worsens by two or more scores, lasting $\geqslant 1$ min. Radial shortening is defined as the decrease in length during systole of an imaginary radius from the endocardium to the center of the ventricular cavity in the midpapillary muscle short-axis cross- section[24] (using reference systems, see below). Myocardial thickening is defined as the increase in the distance between the endocardial and epicardial border during systole on an arbitrary scale of + + + to systolic thinning. Normal value of the left ventricular systolic wall thickening [(systolic wall thickness − diastolic wall thickness)/ systolic wall thickness)] is 0.23–0.35.

In approximately 8–10% of patients a true left ventricular short-axis cross-section view cannot be obtained because of horizontal displacement of the heart by the contents of the abdomen[26] (obesity, ascites, etc.). In such cases a midesophageal longitudinal plane two-chamber view, available with multiplane and biplane probe, can be used. Similarly, transgastric longitudinal plane displays the true apex in majority of cases.

According to the American Society of Echocardiography,[25] the left ventricular long-axis view is divided into three parts (Fig. 7.6). These are termed basal, mid and apical regions. The basal portion extends from the mitral valve annulus to the tips of the papillary muscles; the midportion extends from the tips to the bases of the papillary muscles, and the apical region constitutes the remainder of the ventricle.

The most frequently involved segments in ischemia are those in the midpapillary muscle short-axis image, followed by the apical segment. The midpapillary short axis, therefore, which includes segments of myocardium representing all three major coronary atreries, appears to be the best single view with which to monitor segmental wall motion abnormalities associated with ischemia.[24,26,27] Nevertheless, it should be realized that monitoring only one view necessarily results in a failure to detect wall

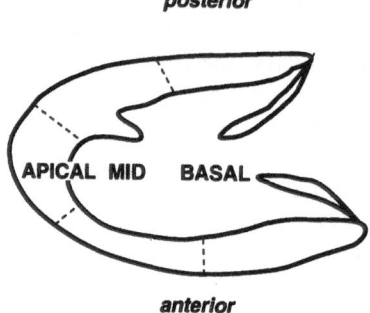

posterior

APICAL MID   BASAL

anterior

Fig. 7.6. Division of the longitudinal plane of the left ventricle into five segments (basal posterior, basal anterior, midposterior, midanterior and apical), as recommended by the American Society of Echocardiography

motion abnormalities that may develop at other levels of the ventricle.[16,26,28,29] If the patient's coronary anatomy is known from coronary angiography, an appropriate level for monitoring segments at risk may be selected.[24,26]

General considerations

Clinical, quantitative real-time examination of two-dimensional images for segmental wall motion abnormalities requires on stop frames systematic, segment-by-segment examination of systolic endocardial motion and wall thickening. When imaged at a short-axis cross-section at the level of the papillary muscle, all myocardial segments of the left ventricle move inward and thicken during systole. In fact, contraction increases from the base to the apex, as described by wall thickening and circumferential shortening of the endocardium. Haendchen et al.[30] found the fractional area change of the left ventricular cavity to be 40% at the base of the heart, increasing to 60% at the apex. Since the diastolic area at the apex is considerably less than that of the base, however, it is still the base of the heart that contributes the most to stroke volume.

The left ventricular septum must be given separate consideration. Although normal septal wall thickening is approximately 30%, it must be realized that this refers to the muscular lower portion of the septum. There is a basal membranous part that does not exhibit the same degree of contraction. Unlike the left ventricular free wall, the septum is also part of the right ventricle and subject to forces from both sides. When the septum is examined in left ventricular short-axis cross-section at the level of the mitral valve, it is normally found to move paradoxically, i.e., whereas left ventricular free wall moves inward during systole, the septum moves outward.

Apart from the normal systolic inward motion and thickening of the left ventricular wall, lateral motion and a small degree of counterclockwise rotation of the whole heart also occur in normal systole.[31-33] Moreover, during the respiratory cycle the heart shifts its position in the thorax independently from the movements described above,[21,32] and it is reasonable to take echocardiographic recordings for reading from the midexpiration phase to eliminate cardiac motion due to respiration. Thus, any wall motion analysis must account not only for the intrinsic centripetal motion ("contractile" motion) of the walls but also for extrinsic or translational and rotational motion of the entire heart.

Once the points that comprise the border are established, their position can be recorded by (a) manual tracing directly from the video screen, (b) digital tracing using an electronically directed cursor, (c) using an automated border-tracing algorithm.

The manual tracing of boundaries directly from the video screen is relatively crude approach, given the precision in measurement required and the parallax errors inherent in any screen-derived measurement. Tracing the boundaries with digital recording of point coordinates is preferred because it removes any parallax error and permits storage of the contours in a form that allows their subsequent reconstruction and manipulation. Because the sampling rate of digitizers is typically constant, while the speed at which the operator can trace the borders, the point density of the digitizer contours will usually be large and the points unevenly spaced. Points used to define the contour, therefore, are typically filtered and the number of points reduced. This initial reduction has a smoothing effect on raw data, which will vary with the type of filtering and the degree of point reduction.

Reference systems

Echocardiographic interpretation of segmental wall motion abnormalities is critically dependent on the reviewer's ability to distinguish between segmental motion of the endocardium resulting from contraction of underlying myocardium and motion generated by the translational and rotational movement of the heart. The reviewer must be able to evaluate the abnormalities in a moving frame of reference that translates and rotates in perfect synchrony with the heart. Because the analysis of systolic wall motion requires a comparison of diastolic and systolic images, the most important step is that the image borders be referenced to a specific "geographic" locations. Taking into account that echocardigraphic image is shown on a two-dimensional screen, the same system of coordinates could be used to describe the movement of single endocardial and epicardial points on the section plane. This approach, simple in concept is, however, strongly limited by the heart's movements in the space irrespective of the dynamic geometry of ventricular contraction.[32]

There are two major categories of reference methods (Fig. 7.7):

(1) those by which myocardial borders are related to some *fixed* point on the video screen i.e., *fixed reference system*, using the boundaries of the video raster (*external*).

(2) those by which the end-systolic image is transposed or floated on the end-diastolic contour, i.e., *floating reference system*, using the references within the heart (*internal*), which works in three different ways:

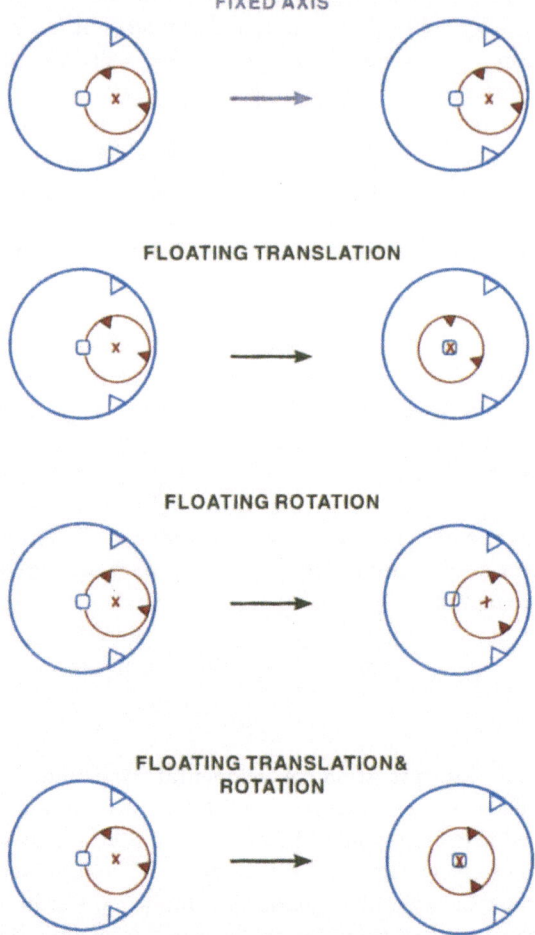

Fig. 7.7. Reference systems. Stylized diagrams of systolic and diastolic borders of the left ventricular short axis, demonstrating the principles of the fixed axis and floating axis reference systems. Outer circle represents diastolic contour and inner circle systolic contour. References points: the two papillary muscles are schematically shown as triangles (open triangles in diastole and closed triangles in systole); X, systolic center of mass; # diastolic center of the mass. Left column schematic shows the translational and rotational movements of the heart and right column shows the results after the corresponding reference analysis is applied

(i) those realigning the end-systolic and end-diastolic contours only by *translation* of one outline over the other by superimposition of indexing points;

(ii) those realigning the end-systolic and end-diastolic contours only by *rotation* of one outline over the other by superimposition of indexing points;

(iii) correcting for both translation and rotation.

Fixed reference system is the simplest reference system which uses the boundaries of the video raster for the alignment of individual frames. In this format, endocardial and epicardial interface position is compared at end-diastole and end-systole.[24] In physicomechanical terms this means a comparison of the end-diastolic and end-systolic contours in their positions relative to the transducer and video screen.[27] For the fixed axis analysis the radii are generated from the midpoint of the diastolic contour, and the systolic radial shortening and systolic wall thickening are calculated,[29,33] *ignoring*[21] the translational and rotational movements of the heart (superimposition of ventricular contours using the margins of the video raster does not permit such correction).

Alternatively, floating reference systems attempt to *control*[21] and to *correct*[24,32–34] for translational and/or rotational movements of the heart. This is performed by superimposing (floating) one or two reference point(s) identified on both the systolic and diastolic images.[24,32] In physicomathematical terms this means that the system is moving together with the heart, so only those movements that really express contraction (not the heart's movement in space) should be evaluated.

For the floating reference system the endocardial tracings are made on a transparent overlay (acetate paper)[33] placed on the monitor screen. After outlining, the end-systolic contour is transposed onto the diastolic one so that the centers or indexing points of each image are exactly superimposed.

Having aligned systolic and diastolic contours using either a fixed axis or floating axis reference system and decided which parameter of regional function is to be measured, it is necessary to choose a method to quantify the extent and severity of abnormal endocardial motion and/or wall thickening. For the left ventricular short axis plane most accepted method is construction of radial chords (Fig. 7.5) between the reference point (center or centroid) and both systolic and diastolic contours if endo-cardial excursion is to be measured or between the centroid and endocardial and epicardial boundaries if wall thickening is to be measured.

Concerning long-axis left ventricular plane most used methods for assessing regional systolic wall motion analysis are construction of the perpendicular chords or combination of perpendicular and radial chords (Fig. 7.8) The major limitation of the perpendicular chord method, therefore, is the high degree of variability in the range of normal apical motion, caused predominately by the sensitivity of the

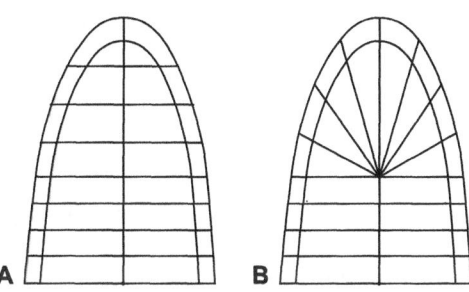

Fig. 7.8. Methods of measuring the extent of wall motion for the left ventricular long-axis view. (A) Series of parallel, evenly placed, chords constructed perpendicular to the long axis of the ventricle. (B) A series of perpendicular chords constructed perpendicular to the long axis of the ventricle, from the base to midventricle, and series of radii constructed from the midpoint of the long axis of the ventricle from the midventricle to apex

algorithm to small changes in position of the midventricular reference line. In an effort to reduce variability in the range of apical motion as assessed from apical images an alternative method has been employed in which a combination of perpendicular and radial chords are constructed between a reference line and the ventricular contours. In this construct, perpendicular chords are used to measure motion at the base of the ventricle, and radial chords are used to measure apical motion (Fig. 7.8B). Although this algorithm reduces the degree of variability in the range of normal motion in the region of the apex and is more sensitive to apical abnormality, it is still limited by the variability encountered when defining the central reference line from which the chords originate and therefore has not been widely used.

Methods for calculating the central reference (centroid) for an individual frame

Unfortunately, there are no true anatomic landmark within the left ventricular cavity that can serve as an internal reference point. Therefore, this point must always be derived. Because all quantitative measurements of endocardial excursion critically depend on the center (centroid, center of the mass) chosen the identification of a reproducible reliable center becomes extremely important. Two general methods have been suggested.

The first defines the central reference as the bisector of a line running from a fixed point on the left ventricular wall (e.g., the posterior junction of the right and left ventricles) to the furthest point on the opposite endocardial surface[35] or the bisector of line running from a fixed external reference (e.g., the midpoint of the inter-ventricular septum) to the opposite free ventricular wall such that it divides the cavity area in half.[36] The accuracy of these bisecting points as centers of reference for radial measurements of ventricular function has not, to date, truly been tested. Although relatively simple to implement, these approaches appear to have several theoretic limitations. First, the bisecting points have no inherent or consistently demonstrated relationship to the true center of the left ventricular tomograms. Second, contraction-induced distortions in ventricular shape will further alter any relationship that exist between arbitrarily derived points and the actual ventricular center; and the effects will vary depending whether the intercepts of the reference line are included in the distortion or not. Moreover, although any derived center by definition will be an approximation, the greater the number of points included in the computation of the reference, the more accurate it should be. Although not specifically tested, the fact that significant difference can be detected between methods, of which calculate the center from large numbers of points, suggests that two-point method should be even less reproducible.

The second general approach is to compute the center of the left ventricle as the center of the region bounded by one of the margins of the left ventricular tomogram. The tomographic two-dimensional echocardiogram provides several anatomic interfaces or areas from which the central reference can be calculated. Likewise, a variety of mathematical methods can be applied to these anatomic data to derive central point. It has been demonstrated[37] that there is significant method-related difference in the reproducibility between observers of the calculated centers, with endocardial based centers being more reproducible than those that use the epicardium.

Centroid calculated as the center of area appear to be more reproducible than those calculated as the center of coordinates. This difference is to be expected because the center of coordinate is the average of all coordinates on the boundary and therefore is sensitive to differences in single coordinates, each of which coordinates equally to the center. The center of area, in contrast, is an integral over the entire region bounded by the epicardial or endocardial margin and therefore should be less sensitive to small changes in coordinates on either boundary.

The validity of the different reference methods has been examined by several investigators. Schnittger et al.[32] studied the use of 44 variations of the different reference methods to compare their accuracy in the quantitation of ventricular wall motion in short-axis cross-section and the long-axis of the left ventricle. The broad categories of reference methods used a fixed external reference, a floating reference correcting for translation, and a floating reference correcting for both translation and rotation. Initially, the left ventricular wall motions of 20 normal subjects were analyzed and plotted to obtain a 95% confidence interval for each of the 44 methods. Subsequently, the wall motions of an additional 10 normal and 31 abnormal subjects were compared with the initial group. This study revealed that the absolute values for left ventricular wall motion varied markedly when different reference methodswere applied to the same two-dimensional view, and also when the same reference method was applied to different views. Fixed external reference systems generally resulted in wider normal bands than did the floating axis method. For each reference method, the band of normal wall motion was wider for a short axis view at the level of the mitral valve than for one at the papillary muscle. The fulcrum of torsion appears to lie in the body of the left ventricle at the midpapillary muscle level. Translational movement was also found to be minimal at this level.

Therefore, a fixed reference analysis method was found to be satisfactory for the short-axis view at the papillary muscle level, and in fact was superior to the floating axis reference system for this view. Sensitivity and specifity for normal wall motion at this level were both 95%, clearly superior to the values obtained with other two-dimensional views. Schnittger's results[32] compare well with the work group of Parisi et al.[35] who, using slightly different methods, found a sensitivity of 95%, specificity of 89%, and predictive accuracy of 92% with fixed reference analysis of the same short-axis view. Actually, the extent of the rotational movement of the heart at the level of the papillary muscles has been found to be only 3°–4° in normal and in patients with various heart diseases.[21] All these results suggest that correction for rotation is unnecessary for short-axis cross-section of the basal two thirds of the heart. This issue has not been examined at the cardiac apex. It seems that rotation hire may be a more significant factor. If so, it will pose a significant problem to quantitative analysis since there are no internal landmarks to which to relate the diastolic and systolic contours.

Several investigators have examined the advantages of dividing the ventricular image into radii vs areas, again usually considering only endocardial borders. It has been demonstrated that predictive accuracy is greater with an area method than with a radial method in conjunction with a fixed reference system.[36,38] When a floating axis reference system was used, however, there was no difference between radial and area methods.

In general, floating reference systems tend to minimize the degree of abnormal motion,[24,39] underestimating or "normalizing"[33] SWMA (Fig. 7.9) and thus may give false-negative observations.[27] On the other hand, the fixed external reference system tends to overestimate SWMA[39] (Fig. 7.9) and may give false-positive results.[27] Given this, is there any theoretical and practical reason to favor one over the other? To answer this question, one must first to determine how much translational and rotational motion occurs in various clinical settings. Practically, however, this is impossible in everyday use of two-dimensional echocardiography. Therefore, controversy over the reference systems remains unresolved and awaits further investigation.[34]

Systolic wall thickening analysis

Quantitative analysis of systolic wall thickening is a major alternative to analyzing endocardial wall motion. It has some important advantages over the latter. Quantification using systolic thickening is felt to be independent of a center of mass and relatively uninfluenced by translation or rotation.[40-42] Endocardial motion may have passive component[40] whereas systolic thickening does not. In addition, the analysis of systolic thickening has sounder experimental support. It has been shown with sonomicrometry that systolic wall thickening correlates closely with subendo-

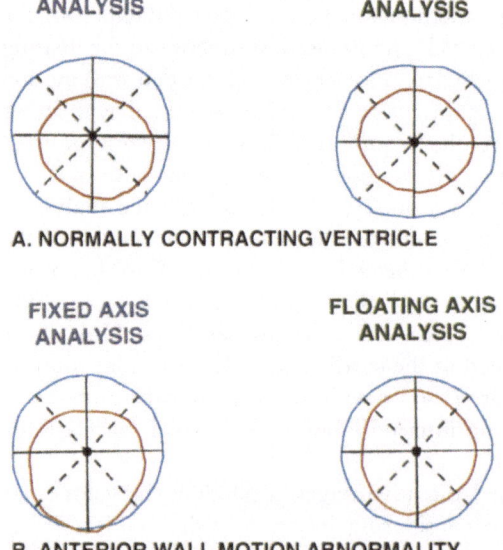

Fig. 7.9. Representation of problems with fixed and floating axis systems. (A) Fixed and floating axis wall motion analyses (area shrinkage) of a *normally contracting ventricle with anterior translation* of the heart. Fixed axis analysis leads to the conclusion that anterior hypo-kinesis is present. Floating axis analysis superimposes the diastolic and systolic centers and normalizes wall motion. (B) Fixed and floating axis analyses of a ventricle *with an anterior wall motion abnormality and no translation* of the heart. Fixed axis analysis correctly localizes the abnormality. Because the center moves toward the wall motion abnormality in systole, super-imposition of the diastolic and systolic centers falsely normalizes anterior endocardial motion

cardial shortening, subendocardial blood flow and transmural blood flow.[21] Moreover, it accurately separates infarcted and noninfarcted tissue.[21] Accordingly,
several studies have shown very good correlation between the extent of abnormal
systolic thickening and infarct size.

However, systolic wall thickening analyses are not without problems. Definition
of the range of normal systolic thickening in different parts of the left ventricle has
the same problems as endocardial motion analysis. Another limitation is that precise
quantitation of the degree of the thinning (epicardial dropout) is not possible.[34] In
addition, the "threshold phenomenon" identified by Lieberman et al.[40] has been
called a potential limitation of systolic wall thickening analysis. They found that as
the transmural extent of ischemia exceeded 20%, systolic thickening deteriorates no
further. This prevents precise "sizing" of tissue infarct size (although not necessarily
the circumferential extent of infarction).

Finally, there are also problems with the system in the analysis of systolic
thickening. Systolic thickening is often measured along radii generated from the
center of mass. It is assumed that these radii will intersect the wall nearly perpendicular to the tangents to endocardium and epicardium. This may not be the
case when contraction is asymmetrical. Moreover, of potentially greater importance
is that all systems reported to date use an analysis that is based on the degree of the
circumference of the left ventricle that is dysfunctional in systole. Fig. 7.10 illustrates

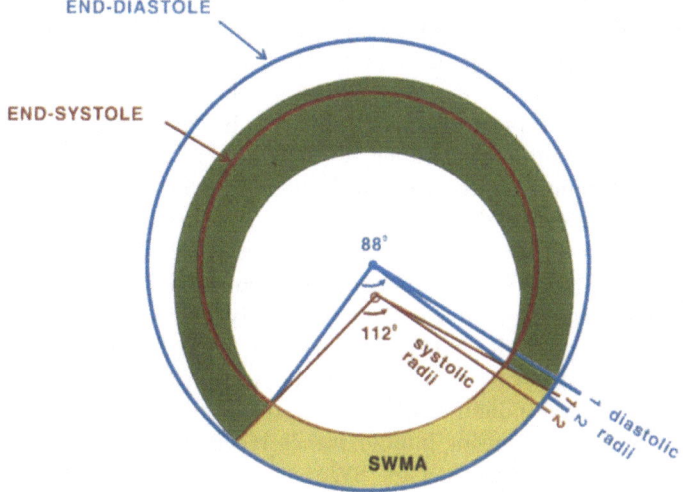

Fig. 7.10. Stylized diagram of a short-axis echocardiographic systolic thickening analysis.
Radii are generated from the centers of mass for the diastolic and systolic contours.
Equivalent radii are determined by their positions on the radial coordinate plot (i.e., diastolic
radius 1 is matched to systolic radius 1) rather than by any myocardial landmark. In the
example, the dysfunctional segment subtends an angle of 88° or 24% of the diastolic
circumference versus 112° or 31% of the systolic circumference. Since diastolic radii 1 and
2 (which intersect abnormally contracting myocardium) show an extent of dysfunction of
31% rather than the 24% predicted from the diastolic image, this method would lead to
overestimation of the dysfunctional region (*SWMA*)

a problem with this approach. In order for radii to intersect the wall correctly, end-diastolic radii for the assessment of end-diastolic thickness are constructed from an end-diastolic centroid, and end-systolic radii for assessment of end-systolic thickness are constructed from an end-systolic centroid. Equivalent radii are determined by their positions on the radial coordinate plot rather than by any myocardial landmark. With asymmetrical contraction, similarly numbered radii will not intersect the same segment of myocardium in systole and in diastole.[21] This process will lead to an overestimation of the extent of dysfunction. Nevertheless, recently, good results using only systolic wall thickening in the evaluation of tran- sient myocardial ischemia have been reported using a nonautomated "eyeball" method.[12,43]

An alternative to the above-mentioned methodological difficulties using fixed or floating reference systems in evaluating systolic wall thickening is the center-wall method.[44] It examines wall thickening in all areas of the myocardium and uses a multistep analytical procedure that requires full visualization of the entire endocardium and epicardium, a condition that may not be the case in all patients.[43] It also requires software that is not universally available in the standard echo instrument calculation packages.

In summary, two-dimensional echocardiographic wall motion and systolic wall thickening analyses compare favorably in terms of reproducibility and accuracy with the older technique of contrast ventriculography. The choice of analysis system (fixed versus floating) and the type of analysis (motion versus thickening) are to some extent arbitrary,[21] but some general conclusions can be drawn. For identification of the presence or absence of a contraction abnormality, either motion or thickening analysis is adequate and both have to be estimated. When two-dimensional images are of very good quality, systolic thickening analysis is superior to wall motion analysis primarily because there is less overlap of adjacent normally contracting myocardium. Consequently, there is less overestimation of ischemic regions with thickening analysis. For wall motion in the left ventricular short-axis cross-section at the level of the papillary muscles, fixed axis analysis may be superior to floating axis, but for the long-axis, floating analysis should be performed.

Clearly, **not all SWMA are indicative of myocardial ischemia** or infarction. Interpretation of septal motion is most frequently confounded by discoordinated contraction. For example, when the septum is viable and nonischemic, it appreciably thickens during systole, although its inward motion can begin slightly before or after inward motion of the other walls of the left ventricle. Furthermore, SWMA can be detected during bundle branch block and ventricular pacing.[21,26]

Another conceivable cause of acute SWMA is the unmasking of areas of scarring by changes in afterload.[24,45] For instance, a marked increase in blood pressure might retard contraction in an already damaged segment of myocardium more than in a normal segment. However, another expert does not accept load dependence of SWMA as a factor that may interfere with evaluation of the wall motion pattern.[26]

The tethering or systolic dysfunction of nonischemic myocardium adjacent to ischemic or infarcted myocardium is also commonly mentioned as another cause of "artifactual" SWMA. Tethering probably accounts for the consistent overestimation of infarct size by two-dimensional echocardiography when compared with that found on postmortem studies. Actually, tethering may help to detect intraoperative myocardial ischemia by making a new SWMA involved in an area of myocardium slightly larger than the true area of ischemia.[27] Tethering does not create new SWMAs in the absence of acute myocardial·ischemia.

Finally, causes of SWMA may also be postischemic myocardial stunning and postcardiac surgery myocardial stunning. What is pathophysiologically stunned myocardium? For approximately four decades after Tennant and Wiggers' classical observation of the effects of coronary occlusion on myocardial contraction[1] it was thought that after severe ischemia myocardium either became irreversibly jeopardized, i.e., infarction developed, or promptly recovered. However, in the 1980s it became clear that after a brief episode of severe ischemia, prolonged dysfunction with gradual return of contractile activity occurred, a condition termed myocardial stunning.[46,47] Myocardial stunning is prolonged but temporary postischemic ventricular dysfunction without necrosis; the stunned myocardium is viable and exhibits contractile reserve. Stunning may occur with demand-induced ischemia, with coronary spasm, and may be limited to the subendocardium.[46] In anesthesia practice, myocardial stunning probably occurs most frequently in the hearts of patients who have cardiac arrest, after successful cardiopulmonary resuscitation, after cardiac arrest during cardiopulmonary bypass[48] or after coronary occlusion during balloon angioplasty.[46] Similarly, it occurs in ICUs after thrombolytic therapy in patients having acute myocardial infarction, and in those with severe ischemia due to coronary vasospasm (Prinzmetal's angina) or unstable angina.[46] The process of amelioration after stunning is called hibernation.[46,47]

Nonischemic causes of abnormal left ventricular wall motion:
— bundle branch block
— ventricular pacing
— prosthetic valve
— image plane throughout membranous septum
— myocarditis and infiltrative disorders of the left ventricle
Particular (specific) causes for SWMA:
— postischemic myocardial stunning
— postcardiac surgery myocardial stunning
In the overwhelming majority of these instances, although endocardial excursion is abnormal, wall thickening will be normal, and this distinction permits the identification of these abnormalities as nonischemic. Focal myocarditis and infiltrative disorders are indistinguishable from myocardial ischemia in that both endocardial excursion and wall thickening are depressed.

Biplane and multiplane TEE imaging

It is clear that ischemia confined to the apex or base of the left ventricle will be missed if only the midpapillary muscle cross-section is monitored.[26,49-53] At the same time, the apex is an extremely important region to evaluate accurately since apical wall motion abnormalities are common with disease of the left anterior descending coronary artery. Hegger et al.[54] correlated regional wall asynergy with the site of myocardial infarction in 37 patients. The most frequently involved segments were those in the midpapillary muscle at the short-axis view, followed by the apical

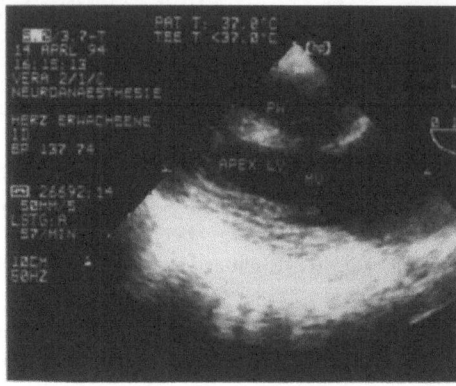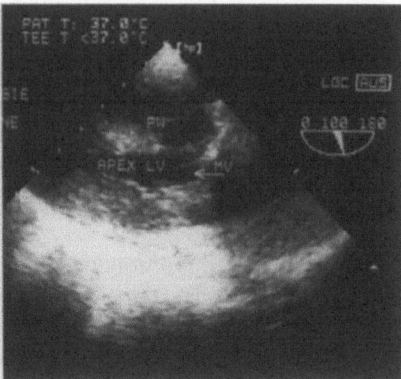

Fig. 7.11. Left ventricular transgastric long-axis view in diastole (left) and systole (right) obtained from a position of the probe for the short-axis at the level of the papillary muscle plane. This view is obtained only by changing the scanning angle from 0° to 100° (see external screen dial). One can appreciate the left ventricular apex. *LV* left ventricle; *MV* mitral valve; *PW* posterior wall

segment. One solution to this problem is to reposition the probe frequently to view other cross-sections, but this is impractical. The multiplane TEE transducer from Howlett Packard makes it possible to obtain a very good view of the apex by use of only a control button (on the echoscope handle), without repositioning the probe[49] (Fig. 7.11). By not moving the probe, the process of monitoring is simplified, the chances of introducing false positives secondary to changes in orientation of the transducer are minimized, and the remote possibility of esophageal trauma is reduced. From mid-esophageal position longitudinal scanning (by means of longitudinal plane probe or rotating multiplane transducer from 0 to 90°) permits also very good assessment of left ventricular apex. The use of biplane TEE monitoring during anesthesia has been reported to increase the sensitivity for detection of severe SWMA by 25%.[49-52]

Analysis of apical wall motion, unfortunately, is the most difficult area of the ventricle to evaluate irrespective of the technique used. With contrast ventriculography, Sheehan et al.[55] found that since the magnitude of motion is low and variability is high at the apex, reliability of motion measurement is worse there than in any other ventricular region. They concluded that motion must be nearly dyskinetic to be abnormal. Other authors[38] did not find high variability to be a significant problem with two-dimensional echocardiography. Further, in the midesophageal transverse views, Erbel et al.[56] showed that the operator-defined echocardiographic apex was often significantly different from the anatomical apex, and thus the apex is often "truncated" by echocardiography. The "truncated" apex may falsely enhance wall motion, which can explain the difficulties in differentiation of abnormal from normal apical motion.

Cine loop and SWMA

In the operating room, the anesthesiologist sometimes must make swift decisions and he does not have time for the described quantitative and semiquantitative scoring systems in the evaluation of ischemia. In such cases, a qualitative interpretation of echocardiographic findings can be used. Clearly, new SWMA can be missed if recall of baseline wall motion is inadequate. *Quad-screen cine loop* systems are commercially available and definitely assist in the recognition of SWMA.[26,49] Biplane real-time imaging is currently not available, but this may be simulated by recording one plane into the cine loop and subsequently displaying it in a side-by-side manner with the second plane using a split-screen format (Fig. 7.12).

Unfortunately, no currently available automated wall motion analysis system has proved adequate for TEE images[26] and anesthesiologists must continue to rely on analysis by experienced observers.[35,36] Even when performed by experts, the analysis of segmental wall motion is subjective.[57] Therefore, in many research studies at least two expert readers review the echocardiograms independently. Other investigators have relied upon the simultaneously interpretation of two readers (consensus interpretations). Although more time consuming than the other approaches, independent interpretation should be performed to minimize the risk of bias.

Both quantitative and semiquantiative TEE analyses, however, are tedious. These methods require knowledge of and expertise in echocardiographic interpretation.[34] The observer must examine each segment in turn for wall

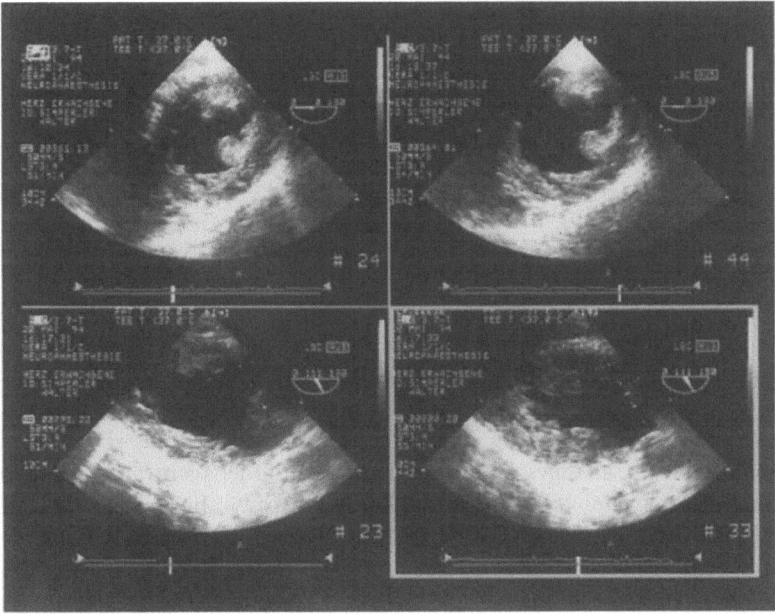

Fig. 7.12. Quad-screen system can be used for intraoperative swift qualitative evaluation of left ventricular wall motion pattern using both transgastric planes. This manner of recording of one plane (short-axis) into cine loop and subsequently displaying it side-by-side with the second plane (long-axis) using a split-screen format simulates biplane real-time imaging. Cine loop permits "recalling of the anesthesiologist's memory" to the earlier patterns of wall motion

thickening and inward motion during systole. In addition, semiquantitative assessment and cine loop on-line can be subjective if the observer does not adhere to strict guidelines established for regional wall motion analysis. Accuracy and consistency of echocardiographic interpretation require frequent determination of both intraobserver and interobserver variability. A study by Saada et al.[58] examined the validity of two-dimensional evaluation of TEE. Anesthesia residents (with minimal TEE experience) and faculty anesthesiologists (with experience in more than 50 cases) were asked to evaluate intraoperative SWMA. The TEE short-axis views were simultaneously recorded on videotapes for subsequent evaluation by two independent, experienced observers. Residents correctly identified 97% of normal wall motion, and faculty members, 98%. Of the segments with abnormal wall motion detected by expert readers, residents were able to detect 61% and faculty members, 77%. The experienced readers disagreed on 5% of the segments (normal versus mild hypokinesia). Three episodes of ischemia (change of grade greater than or equal to 2) were detected by the expert readers; one was detected by the faculty members and none by the residents. Thus, even trained observers can miss intraoperative ischemic events. Two-dimensional intraoperative use of TEE for accurately detecting ischemia therefore is complex and requires a significant amount of echocardiographic training.[34]

Methodological problems

— The investigator must be able to distinguish myocardial contraction from motion that is due to translation and rotation of the whole heart and spatial movement of the heart during respiration. Using either system is complicated because of the limitations of each (capacity for both false-positive and false-negative diagnoses) and is time consuming.
— "On-line" interpretation is less sensitive than "off-line" examination.
— Qualitative interpretation is less sensitive than quantitative assessment.
— The contraction pattern of the normal left ventricle is not simply concentric and uniform. Myocardial systolic shortening and cross-sectional fractional area change, as seen by two-dimensional echo, increase from the mitral valve (38%) to the lower LV level (60%). Interventricular septal segments exhibit lowest contraction at the base, but increase from base to apex. Lateral regions do not show significant changes along the length of the left ventricle. These regional differences may not be essential in assessing grossly abnormal contraction, but could be critical for the interpretation of hypokinesis, as is frequently encountered in patients with CAD.
— Nonischemic causes of regional wall motion abnormalities.
— No uniform agreement over the criteria of dysfunctional myocardium; hypokinesis is sensitive but not specific.
— Influence of changes in afterload, i.e., load dependence.
— Tethering effect caused by neighboring infarcted segments.
— Monitoring a single-short axis view during anesthesia may miss myocardial ischemia localized outside the scanning plane.

—Because monitoring by TEE is uncomfortable for the awake patient, TEE is impractical for use before the induction of anesthesia and in the postoperative period, both of which represent high-risk periods for the development of myocardial ischemia. Alternatively, the transthoracic approach can be used, which requires more skill.

References

1. Tennant R, Wiggers C. The effect of coronary occlusion on myocardial contraction. Am J Physiol 112: 351–361, 1935
2. Forrester JS, Wyatt HL. Functional significance of regional ischemic contraction abnormalities. Circulation 54: 64–71, 1976
3. Waters DD, da Luz P, Wyatt HL, Swan HLC, Forrester JS. Early changes in regional and global left ventricular function induced by graded reduction in regional coronary perfusion. Am J Cardiol 39: 537–543, 1977
4. Tomoike H, Franklin D, Ross J Jr. Detection of myocardial ischemia by regional dysfunction during and after rapid pacing in conscious dogs. Circulation 58: 48–56, 1978
5. Battler A, Froelicher VF, Gallagher KP. Dissociation between regional myocardial dysfunction and ECG changes during ischemia in the conscious dog. Circulation 62: 735–739, 1980
6. Hauser AM, Gangadharan V, Ramos RG. Sequence of mechanical, electro-cardiographic and clinical effects of repeated coronary artery occlusion in human beings: echocardio- graphic observation during coronary angioplasty. J Am Coll Cardiol 5: 193–205, 1985
7. Wohlgelernter D, Cleman M, Highman H. Regional myocardial dysfunction during coronary angioplasty: evaluation by two-dimensional echocardiography and 12-lead electrocardiography. J Am Coll Cardiol 7: 1245–1249, 1986
8. Smith JS, Cahalan MK, Benefiel DJ, Byrd BF, Lurz FW, Shapiro WA, Roizen MF, Bouchard A, Schiller NB. Intraoperative detection of myocardial ischemia in high-risk patients: electrocardiography versus two-dimensional transesophageal echocar-diography. Circulation 72: 1015–1021, 1985
9. Abel MD, Nishimura RA, Callahan MJ, Rehder K, Ilstrup DM, Taijik J. Evaluation of intraoperative transesophageal two-dimensional echocardiography. Anesthesiology 66: 64–68, 1987
10. Leung JM, O'Kelly B, Browner WS, Tubau J, Hollenberg M, Mangano DT, SPI Research Group. Prognostic importance of postbypass regional wall motion abnormalities in patients undergoing coronary artery bypass graft surgery. Anesthesiology 71: 16–25, 1989
11. Leung JM, O'Kelly BF, Mangano DT, SPI Research group. Relationship of regional wall motion abnormalities to hemodynamic indices of myocardial oxygen supply and demand in patients undergoing CABG surgery. Anesthesiology 73: 802–814, 1990
12. Voici P, Bilotta F, Aronson S, Scibilia G, Caretta Q, Mercanti C, Marino B, Thisted R, Roizen MF, Reale A. Echocardiographic analysis of dysfunctional and normal myo-cardial segments before and immediately after coronary artery bypass graft surgery. Anesth Analg 75: 213–218, 1992
13. Owal A, Echrenberger J, Brodin A. Myocardial ischaemia as judged from transesophagealechocardiography and ECG in the early phase after coronary artery bypass surgery. Acta Anaesth Scand 37: 92–96, 1993
14. Harris SN, Gordon MA, Urban MK, O'Konor TZ, Barash PG. The pressure rate quotient is not an indicator of myocardial ischemia in humans. An echocardiographic study. Anesthesiology 78: 242–250, 1993

15. Roizen MF, Beapue NP, Alpert RA. Monitoring with two-dimensional transesophageal echocardiography. J Vasc Surg 1: 300–307, 1984
16. Rafferty T. Intraoperative monitoring of ischemia and systolic cardiac function. In: Missiri J, ed. Transesophageal echocardiography. Clinical and intraoperative applications. Churchill Livingstone, New York, p 184, 1993
17. London MJ, Tubau JF, Wong MG, Layug E, Mangano DT. The "natural history" of segmental wall motion abnormalities detected by intraoperative transesophageal echocardiography: A clinically blinded, prospective approach (Abstr). Anesthesiology 69: A79, 1988
18. Hollenberg M, Mangano DT, Browner WS, London MJ, Tubau JF, Tateo IM, SPI Research Group. Predictors of postoperative myocardial ischemia in patients undergoing noncardiac surgery. JAMA 268: 205–209, 1992
19. Fleischer LA, Rosenbaum SH, Nelson AH, Barash PG. The predictive value of perioperative silent ischemia for postoperative ischemic cardiac events in vascular and nonvascular surgery. Am Heart J 122: 980–986, 1991
20. Raby KE, Barry J, Creager MA, Cook F, Weisberg MC, Goldman L. Detection and significance of intraoperative and postoperative myocardial ischemia in peripherial vascular surgery. JAMA 268: 222–227, 1992
21. Force TL, Parisis AF. Quantitative methods for analyzing regional systolic function with two-dimensional echocardiography. In: Kerber RE, ed. Echocardiography in coronary artery disease. Futura, Mount Kisko, p 193, 1988
22. Nishimura RA, Reeder GS, Miller FA. Prognostic value of predischarge 2-dimensional echocardiography after acute myocardial infarction. Am J Cardiol 53: 429–434, 1984
23. Bhatnagar SK, Moussa MAA, Al-Yusut G. The role of prehospital discharge two-dimensional echocardiography in determining the prognosis of survivors of the first myocardial infarction. Am Heart J 109: 472–476, 1985
24. Clements FM, de Bruijn NP. Perioperative evaluation of regional wall motion by transesophageal two-dimensional echocardiography. Anesth Analg 66: 249–261, 1987
25. Schiller N, Shah P, Crawford M, DeMaria A, Devereux R, Feigenbaum H, Gutgesell H, Reichek N, Sahn D, Schnittiger I, Silverman NH. Recommendations for quantification of the left ventricle by two-dimensional echocardiography. J Am Soc Echocard 2: 358–367, 1989
26. Cahalan MK. Intraoperative monitoring for myocardial ischemia with two-dimensional echocardiography. Anesth Cin North Am 9: 581–590, 1991
27. Van Daele MERM, Roelandt JRTC. Intraoperative monitoring. In: Sutherland GR, Roelandt JRTC, Fraser A, Anderson RH, eds. Transesophageal echocardiography in clinical practice. Cower, London, New York, pp 12.1–12.9, 1991
28. Stanley TE. Quantitative echocardiography. In: deBruijn NP, Clements FM, eds. Intraoperative use of echocardiography. Lippincott, Philadelphia, pp 77–91, 1991
29. Huemer G, Kolev N, Zimpfer M. Comparisons of Doppler transmitral diastolic parameters and systolic wall motion abnormalities during perioperative ischemia (Abstr). Anesthesiology 81: A107, 1994
30. Haendchen RV, Wyatt Hl, Maurer J, Zwehl W, Baer M, Merbaum S, Corday E. Quantitation of regional cardiac function by two-dimensional echocardiography. I. Pattern of contraction in the normal left ventricle. Circulation 67: 1234–1245, 1983
31. Huemer G, Kolev N, Kurz A, Zimpfer M. Influence of positive end-expiratory pressure on right and left ventricular performance assessed by Doppler two-dimensional echocardiography. Chest 106: 67–73, 1994
32. Schnittger I, Fitzgerald PJ, Gordon EP, Alderman EL, Popp RL. Computerized quantitative analysis of left ventricular wall motion by two-dimensional echocardiography. Circulation 70: 242–254, 1984
33. Force T, Bloomfeld P, O'Boyle JE, Khuri SF, Josa M, Parisis AF. Quantitative two-dimensional echocardiographic analysis of regional wall motion in patients with perioperative myocardial infarction. Circulation 70: 233–241, 1984

34. Leung JM, Schiller NB, Mangano DT. Assessment of left ventricular function using two-dimensional echocardiography. In: deBrujin NP, Clements FM. Intraoperative use of echocardiography. Lippincott, Philadelphia, pp 59–74, 1991

35. Parisi AF, Moynihan PF, Folland ED, Feldman CL. Quantitative detection of regional left ventricular contraction abnormalities by two-dimensional echocardiography. II. Accuracy in coronary artery disease. Circulation 63: 761–767, 1981

36. Pandin NC, Kerber RE. Two-dimensional echocardiography in experimental coronary stenosis. I. Sensitivity and specificity in detecting transient myocardial dyskinesis: Comparison with sonomicrometers. Circulation 66: 597–601, 1982

37. Pearlman JD. Echocardiographic definition of the left ventricular centroid: I. Analysis of methods for centroid calculation from a single tomogram. J Am Coll Cardiol 19: 993–999, 1990

38. Moynihan PF, Parisis AF, Feldman CL. Quantitative detection of regional left ventricular contraction abnormalities by two-dimensional echocardiography. I. Analysis of methods. Circulation 63: 752–760, 1981

39. Ihra G, Bacher A, Kolev N, Huemer G, Illievich UM, Spiss CK. Effect of hypothermia (32° C body temperature) on left ventricular systolic wall motion during neurosurgery (Abstr). Anesthesiology 81: A250, 1994

40. Lieberman AN, Weiss JL, Jugdutt. Two-dimensional echocardiography and infarct size: relationship of regional wall motion and thickening to the extent of myocardial infarction in dogs. Circulation 63: 739–743, 1981

41. Lima JAC, Becker LC, Melin JA. Impaired thickening of nonischemic myocardium during acute regional ischemia in dogs. Circulation 71: 1048–1054, 1985

42. Fedel F, Penco M, Dagianti A. Quantification of left ventricular regional wall thickening in two-dimensional echocardiography. Analysis of a new semiautomated method. J Cardiovasc Ultras 4: 201–206, 1985

43. Konstandt SN, Abrahams HP, Nejat M, Reich DL. Are wall thickening measurements reproducible? Anesth Analg 78: 619–623, 1994

44. Sheechan FH, Feneley MP, DeBruijn NP. Quantitative analysis of regional wall. thickening by transesophageal echocardiography. J Thorac Cardiovasc Surg 103: 347–354, 1992

45. Kavanaugh KM, Brenner HM, Gallagher KP, Buda AJ. Effects of afterloads on the functional border zone measured with two-dimensional echocardiography during acute coronary occlusion. Am Heart J 116: 942–953, 1988

46. Braunwald E, Sobel BE. Coronary blood flow and myocardial ischemia. In: Braunwald E, ed. Heart disease. 4th ed. WB Saunders, Philadelphia, pp 1176–1178, 1992

47. Kolev N, Zimpfer M. Impact of ischemia on diastolic function: Clinical relevance and recent Doppler echocardiographic insights. Eur J Anaesth (in press), 1994

48. Braunwald E. The stunned myocardium: Newer insights into mechanisms and clinical applications. J Thorac Cardiovasc Surg 100: 310–315, 1990

49. Kolev N, Ihra G, Leitner K, Spiss CK, Zimpfer M. Improved detection of perioperative myocardial ischemia with multiplane (Hewlett Packard) transesophageal scanning: Two-dimensional biplane and transmitral Doppler echocardiography. J Cardiovasc Diag Proc (NY) (in press), 1994

50. Rouine-Rapp K, Cahalan MK, Ionesku P, Muhiudeen I, Foster E. Detection of wall motion abnormalities: Biplane transesophageal echocardiography vs multiplane transverse cross sections (Abstr). Anesthesiology 77: A481, 1992

51. Shah PM, Kyo S, Matsumura M, Omoto R. Utility of biplane transesophageal echocardiography in left ventricular wall motion analysis. J Cardiothorac Vasc Anesth 5: 316–319, 1991

52. Chung F, Seyone C, Rakowski H. Transesophageal echocardiography may fail to diagnose perioperative myocardial infarction. Can J Anaesth 38: 98–101, 1991

53. Koide Y, Long T, Nomura T, Oka Y. Efficacy of biplane TEE in detecting regional wall motion abnormalities in patients undergoing coronary artery bypass graft (Abstr). Anesthesiology 79: A71, 1993

54. Hegger JJ, Weyman AL, Wann LS, Dilon JC, Feigenbaum H. Cross sectional echocardio- graphy in acute myocardial infarction: detection and localization of regional left ventricular asynergy. Circulation 60: 531–538, 1979
55. Sheehan FH, Steward AK, Dodge HT. Variability in the measurement of regional left ventricular wall motion from contrast angiogram. Circulation 68: 550–559, 1983
56. Erbel R, Schweizer P, Lamberz H. Echoventriculography—A simultaneous analysis of two-dimensional echocardiography and cineventriculography. Circulation 67: 205–209, 1983
57. Cahalan MC, Lurz FC, Schiller NB. Transesophageal two-dimensional echocardiographic evaluation of anaesthetic effects on left ventricular function. Br J Anaesth 60: 99S–106S, 1988
58. Saada M, Cahalan MK, Lee E, Schiller NB. Real-time evaluation of segmental wall motion abnormalities (Abstr). Anesth Analg 68: S242, 1989

Automated on-line wall motion analysis

Introduction

Transesophageal two-dimensional echocardiography has emerged as a very good noninvasive technique for studying the mechanical consequences of acute myocardial ischemia: because of its high spatial resolution, its sampling frequency and its safety, wall motion abnormalities can be identified within seconds of onset of ischemia and monitored sequentially.[1-3] The clinical significance of the technique's capability is demonstrated by the close relationship between the extent of the mechanical impairment as evaluated by TEE and the prognosis for patients in whom perioperative ischemia is present.[3-6]

In light of such marvelous characteristics, great efforts have been made to achieve quantitatively accurate evaluations of the segmental wall motion abnormalities (SWMA) visualized by TEE. In a desire to quantitate such abnormalities, multiple computer-based models for wall motion analysis have been developed. We should revise the technique put forward in echocardiography for automated quantitative wall motion abnormalities. Although there are rigorous studies on this subject, the ultimate aim of automated SWMA assessment has still not been achieved definitely.

The most important precondition for automated quantitative wall motion analysis that the image be obtained with appropriate resolution. Partly this depends on the echocardiographic system of image representation. The echocardiographic scan converter, which transforms the analog signal from the transducer into a digital signal, has its own operative speed, which varies from system to system, as well as its own speed for updating the image. This means that for any given time unit, a part of the image collected in the converter is being continually updated, with the result that overall data making up the signal image are never really contemporaneous.

Apart from the technical problems mentioned above, other factors of ananatomical-physiological nature exist that have so far created problems in analyzing the images. The contracting heart makes movements in space (counterclockwise rotation in longitudinal axis and translational in the anterolateral) that could bring about the same echocardiographic section visualizing different anatomic sections during the course of the cardiac cycle.

Principles of border identification

The systolic shortening of the intracavitary radius and thickening of the ventricular wall can in theory be "measured" but for each of them a hypothetical "measurement" creates different technical problems. The first and most important is the identification of the endocardium. It can be done by the operator (by hand) or automated[7] by means of a process that is made up essentially of four steps:[8]

— image enhancement;
— utilization of an algorithm called "edge operator," which determines pixel by pixel what belongs to the endocardial image;

— filling of the space between the pixels definitively attributed to the endocardium to construct its continuous edge;
— elimination of the pixels individually and wrongly attributed to the endocardium.

After the endocardium has been identified it is necessary to record the position of the single points. These two steps (endocardial identification and point of reference) are conceptually distinct yet tend to be identified in most procedures that envisage the continuous or discrete digitilization of the endocardial points by means of electronic cursor or automatic algorithms. The digital recording of the single endocardial points is important since it is precisely on these data (made up of a pair of coordinates that identify on the plane the endocardial point in question) that all the calculations for the quantitative definition of kinesis will subsequently be made.

Principles of the internal "centroid" reference systems

Bearing in mind the circular shape of the cross-section short-axis view of the heart, all the internal systems devised are based on the hypothetical calculation of the ventricular mass, termed "centroid." Fig. 7.13 demonstrates the principle of such quantitative approaches in schematic form superimposed on the left ventricular cross-section short-axis. On the left is a diastolic image. After digitation, the computer determines a mathematical centroid from which multiple radial lines are derived. Any number of equidistant radial lines may be determined around the circumference of the ventricle. Some programs may have as many as 360 such lines. In this example, however, only three lines are shown for simplicity's sake.

The process is repeated in systole (right panel) and the center of the ventricle is calculated once again. For the purposes of deriving a wall motion number, the computer then superimposes the diastolic and systolic centers of the ventricle and compares the position of the endocardium between the two cardiac cycles along each of the radial lines. The resultant number may be expressed as an absolute distance. More commonly, such numbers are expressed as percent shortening.

Fig. 7.13 shows an ideal model in which the center of the ventricle remains the same in systole so that the percent wall motion in the affected segment becomes

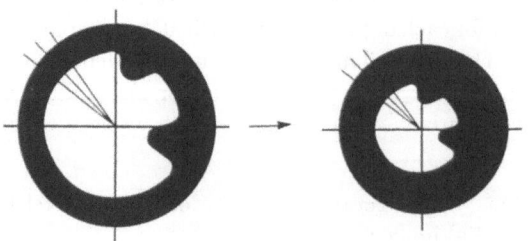

Fig. 7.13. Stylized diagram of the left ventricular short-axis demonstrating normal pattern of diastolic (left) and systolic (right) contours during cardiac cycle

negative (or away from the center). Data derived in such a way are compared to normals and the descriptive indices derived. This example is, however, only ideal. In reality, there are complex spatial differences between the position of the left ventricle in diastole, compared to its position in systole. In normal hearts, the ventricle moves somewhat anteriorly as the whole heart empties. At the same time, there are various rotations about the theoretical centroid of the ventricle, making spatial determination of the true center difficult.

This problem confounds the ability to easily quantify wall movement in individuals with severe wall motion abnormalities induced by acute ischemia. Fig. 7.14 demonstrates one of these significant limitations. In the computer the center of the ventricle is mathematically calculated from the diastolic circumference of the endocardial border. The systolic endocardial border is irregular due to segmental wall motion abnormalities. The calculated systolic centroid, therefore, is profoundly affected and shows displacement upward and to the left. Thus, any computer-derived index of wall motion is then distorted by the abnormality in the systolic configuration of the ventricle. In this example, abnormal percent thickening would be identified by the computer around the entire circumference of the ventricle and the specific abnormality missed. This model for determining the diastolic and systolic center of the ventricle from a mathematical computation of the traced endocardial border is applicable only to very diffusely and symmetrically dilated left ventricles where there is little movement about any axis from the calculated diastolic ventricular center.

Recognition of these limitations has lead to the development of other methods for determination of the ventricular center. One such method depends upon tracing both the diastolic and systolic endocardial and epicardial borders. Left ventricular spatial mass is then calculated and the center of mass derived. While spatial distortions are somewhat reduced with this approach, they still exist to such a degree to that this method is deemed unacceptable.[9]

Other models have been developed in an attempt to overcome these problems. The center of the ventricle has been calculated spatially relating the positions of the ventricle in diastole and systole to that of the chest wall and correcting these positions by the distance from the aorta to the chest wall at the same time in the cardiac cycle. Still other methods depend upon determination of the position of the papillary muscles in diastole and systole and then assuming a ventricular center from these positions. All methods derived from the ventricular centroid suffer from

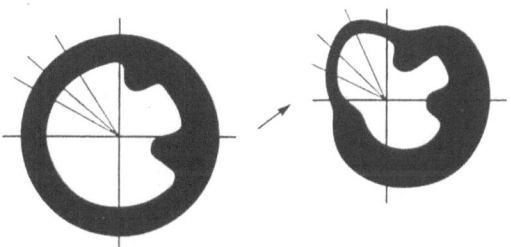

Fig. 7.14. Stylized diagram of the left ventricular short-axis showing a severe limitation of any quantitative model. The center of the ventricle during systole has moved, making quantification unreliable. For more details see text

the complex spatial movements of the heart and all should be criticized in the context of their inability to adequately compensate for such movements.

Wall motion versus wall thickening

Given these limitations, other models of wall thickening rather than percent shortening have been developed. One such method is the "coordinateless" center-line method. In this system, radii are not generated from some derived center point. Instead, a line is generated midway between the end-diastolic and end-systolic contours and then 100 chords are constructed perpendicular to this line (Fig. 7.15). Wall motion is assessed as the length of these chords. The computer then calculates (following the procedure "analysis of the closed loop") the center of the wall thickness along each equidistant point, and each point is connected by a line,[10] thus the name "center-line." The distances between two contours are normalized (i.e., divided) by the length of the end-diastolic contour. More importantly, motion is absolute and can be more reliably compared from region to region than when referenced to an end-diastolic radius or area and expressed as a percent change. This method attempts to overcome several spatial distortions but is not completely free of such problems.[9] Moreover, the center-line method prevents the tangential intersection of radii with endocardium, which may give a false impression of the extent of motion in a region.[11]

Conclusion

The automated quantitative assessment of wall motion abnormalities shown by two-dimensional echocardiography is a very attractive topic because of its potential clinical application in the operating room and ICU. However, even today, it has not been proved that automated quantitative evaluations are better than subjective quantitative or semi-quantitative ones. The capacity of the human eye to integrate in time and space can be emulated by means of complex algorithms that require the use of sophisticated programs and operations. The lateral TEE two-dimensional resolution is still not sufficiently high to obtain reliable results with such methods. The ever-improving resolution, the development of digital echocardiography and of ever more powerful computers for processing images should all contribute to fulfilling our expectations in the near future.

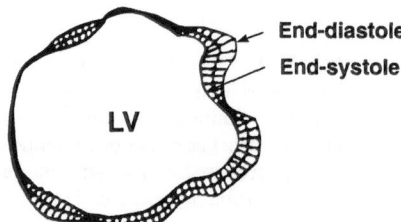

Fig. 7.15. Schematic representation of center-line automated method. End-diastolic and end-systolic contours of left ventricualr short-axis cross-section are given by the chords constructed perpendicular to the centerline. *LV* left ventricle

References

1. Voci P, Billotta S, Aronson S, Scibilia G, Caaretta Q, Mercanti C, Marino B, Thisted R, Roizen MF, Reale A. Echocardiographic analysis of dysfunctional and normal myocardialsegments before and immediately after coronary artery bypass graft surgery. Anesth Analg 75: 213–218, 1992
2. Owall A, Ehrenberg J, Brodin LA. Myocardial ischemia as judged from transoesophageal echocardiography and ECG in the early phase after coronary artery bypass surgery. Acta Anaesth Scand 37: 92–96, 1993
3. Clements FM, de Bruijn NP. Perioperative evaluation of regional wall motion by transesophageal two-dimensional echocardiography. Anesth Analg 66: 249–261, 1987
4. Harris SN, Gordon MA, Urban MK, O'Konor TZ, Barash PG. The pressure rate quotient is not an indicator of myocardial ischemia in humans. An echocardiographic study. Anesthesiology 78: 242–250, 1993
5. Cahalan M. Intraoperative monitoring for myocardial ischemia with two-dimensional echocardiography. Anesth Clin North Am 9: 581–590, 1991
6. Leung JM, O'Kelly BF, Mangano DT, SPI Research Group. Relationship of regional wall motion abnormalities to hemodynamic indices of myocardial oxygen supply and demand in patients undergoing CABG surgery. Anesthesiology 73: 802–814, 1990
7. Bosch JG, Reiber JNC, van Burken G. Developments towards real time frame-to-frame automatic contour detection on echocardiograms. In: Computers in cardiology. Proc 16th Computers in Cardiology Meeting, Long Beach, CA, pp 435–438, 1990
8. Mulleneers RGA, Cheriex EC, Dassen WRM, Beleijlevens BB, Wellens Hjj, Meester GT. The cardiac echostorage and retrieval network system. In: Computers in cardiology. Proc 16th Computers in Cardiology Meeting, Long Beach, CA, pp 211–217, 1990
9. Kisslo J, Sheikh KH. Assessment of wall motion by two-dimensional echocardiography. Should it be qualitative? In: Iliceto S, Rizzon P, Roelandt JRTC, eds. Ultrasound in coronary artery disease. Kluwer, Dordrecht, pp 15–20, 1991
10. Bosch HG, Reiber JHC, van Burken G, Gerbrands JJ, Roelandt JRTC. Automated contour detection on short axis transesophageal echocardiography. In: Erbel R, ed. Transesophageal echocardiography. Springer, Berlin Heidelberg, pp 253–259, 1989
11. Force LT, Parisi AF. Quantitative methods for analyzing regional systolic function with two-dimensional echocardiography. In: Kerber RE, ed. Echocardiography in coronary artery disease. Futura, Mount Kisko, pp 193–220, 1988

Myocardial ischemia and Doppler transmitral diastolic flow

Acute myocardial ischemia is a symptom with multiple pathophysiological mechanisms and varied therapeutic options. Many signs and symptoms of heart dysfunction and pulmonary congestion may relate more directly to the diastolic or *lusitropic* state of the ventricle than to the inotropic state.[1] From a scientific perspective and perhaps from a prognostic standpoint, the precise mechanism underlying the changes in diastolic function is of interest and may be very important. The exact contribution of diastolic dysfunction to morbidity and mortality in coronary artery disease (CAD) patients undergoing cardiac and noncardiac surgery and its relationship to systolic dysfunction, however, remains to be defined. Understanding the significance of diastolic function may seem overwhelming to the basic scientist as well as to the clinician. Rather than being a simple, passive process, diastolic function involves dynamic elements that are closely related to systolic function.[1]

Diastolic function may be defined as the ability of the ventricle to receive an adequate volume while maintaining low intracavitary pressure throughout a wide range of loading conditions and heart rates.[1] To accomplish this, the ventricle relaxes during early diastole and the walls distend readily, allowing the chamber to receive a wide range of inflow volumes at a low filling pressure. To ensure optimal diastolic filling, the left atrium contracts before ventricular activation, providing an additional boost to ventricular filling.

From a physiological standpoint, ventricular diastolic function has been divided into *two components:*[2]

— ventricular relaxation;
— myocardial stiffness.

For clinical purposes, diastole has classically been divided into *four phases:*[2]

1. isovolumic relaxation phase;
2. early rapid filling phase;
3. slow filling phase (diastasis);
4. atrial contraction phase or late diastolic phase.

Ventricular relaxation is one of the most important determinants of left ventricular filling.[3] It is the process by which the myocardium returns to its initial length and tension. The time course of this process is determined by several factors, including active biochemical processes (requiring the removal of cytoplasmatic calcium by sarcoplasmic reticulum), loading conditions and nonuniformity in myocardial relaxation. Relaxation encompasses the end of moyocardial shortening, the isovolumic relaxation period and the rapid filling phase. The relaxation phase occurs after the mitral valve opens, when rapid inflow is a function of the continuing myocardial relaxation. It is known that myocardial muscle is stiffer during action, i.e., during systole. This implies that when the duration of contraction is prolonged or nonuniform, the myocardium may still be in an active state during early diastole and thus stiffer than normal. Ventricular relaxation is best described by isovolumic relaxation indices (negative peak dP/dt, isovolumic relaxation period and the time constant of myocardial relaxation, τ) as well as Doppler transmitral early peak flow.

Chamber stiffness is defined as a change in pressure relative to a change in chamber volume ($\Delta P/\Delta V$); its reciprocal is referred to as compliance (Fig. 4.2). Myocardial stiffness represents the resistance to myocardial stretching during the filling period. It has been argued that left ventricular chamber stiffness, in addition to myocardial stiffness, also reflects the changes in factors extrinsic to left ventricular myocardium, such as loading conditions of the right ventricle, effect of pericardium, pleural pressure and coronary perfusion.[4]

Because the evaluation of diastolic function requires an understanding of the interrelation of ventricular filling volume to pressure ($\Delta V/\Delta P$), Doppler has an advantage over other noninvasive methods (for example, two-dimensional index negative peak dA/dt) for assessing diastolic function, providing nearly direct access to filling pressure. Over the past five years, the relation of the transmitral velocity recorded with pulsed Doppler echocardiography to the filling dynamics of the left ventricle has been extensively studied in health and disease states. Although left ventricular pressures are not available, the mitral inflow velocity is dependent directly on pressure flow interaction, and thus, it can be used to assess changes in filling pressures.

The pressure-volume relationship during diastasis and late diastole is governed by elastic myocardial properties and reflects the interaction between the force resisting the resulting stretching that exists within the myocardium and external forces. Whereas early filling reflects more the changes in active relaxation, diastasis and late diastolic filling are more closely related to passive chamber stiffness.[5]

Recording techniques and parameters of Doppler transmitral inflow

TEE Doppler transmitral inflow velocity is recorded within the midesophageal long-axis four-chamber view or (in some subjects) transgastric long-axis view. In the first case the amplitudes are negative (away from the transducer) and in the latter case are positive (towards the transducer). The transmitral diastolic flow velocity waveforms can be measured at different levels within the mitral valve apparatus by changing the position of the pulsed wave Doppler sample volume, and the waveforms are dependent on the sample volume position. As the mitral valve is somewhat funnel-shaped, the velocities increase progressively across the mitral valve apparatus towards the outlet of the mitral orifice. The ratio of the early rapid filling (E) to late diastolic or atrial (A) filling progressively increases when the sample volume is positioned closer to the outlet of the mitral orificie.[6] The position of a sample volume (which has a 3–5 mm length) in relation to the mitral valve should be observed in a real time to ensure that it remains within the annulus during diastole. The recording should include several cardiac cycles (in the case of time-interval measurements, a speed of 100 mm/sec is recommended). For reasons of intrapatient reproducibility, all pulsed Doppler measurements of the transmitral inflow should be made with the same sample volume in the same position in a given person. One exception exists, namely, when the purpose of measurements is

Doppler-derived isovolumic relaxation time; the sample volume is placed at the left ventricular outflow but in the proximity to the anterior leaflet to record both inflow and outflow signals.[1,7-9] Once again, this intermediate position must be used only for isovolumic relaxation time measurement.

As pointed out earlier flow velocity profiles recorded by the continuous wave Doppler technique represent the highest velocities occurring anywhere the Doppler ultrasound beam. As such they do not reflect the filling pattern of the ventricle as accurately as those obtained by the pulsed Doppler technique, which records the flow velocities at one specific level.

When using the transesophageal approach, the midesophageal four-chamber views required for the accurate recording of transmitral flow velocities as the direction of the inflow jet generally points toward the apex. Little information is available on the differences in transmitral flow velocities obtained from midesophageal long-axis and transgastric left ventricular long-axis view. Any differences is expected to exist, because deviation of the Doppler ultrasound beam from the true direction of blood flow in any one view is likely to be significant. As discussed in chapter 2, angle correction of Doppler flow velocities is performed by dividing the recorded velocities by the cosine of the angle between the Doppler ultrasound beam and the actual direction of blood flow.

The normal transmitral Doppler diastolic flow pattern has two filling waves: the E wave in *early* diastole, and the smaller A wave in late diastole resulting from *atrial* contraction. Fig. 7.16 diagramatically illustrates the Doppler transmitral inflow and left ventricular outflow, which are measured to *assess left ventricular diastolic function*. They can be divided into five categories:

a) absolute velocities, cm/sec;
b) areas under the peaks, i.e., time-velocity integrals, cm;
c) time intervals of cardiac cycle, msec;
d) rate of the slopes of the peak, m/sec^2;
e) ratios of peaks, areas or time intervals, units.

In our experience, the measurement the anesthesiologist needs in the operating room for detecting ischemia is the ratio of peak early diastolic filling to peak atrial filling (E/A). This parameter appears instantaneously on-line. All other parameters, of course, are important and cannot be substituted for E/A ratio, but they are for off-line estimation.[1]

Normal reference values derived from healthy subjects without mitral valvular diseases (aged 45–55 years) are listed in Table 7.7. It has been shown that the majority of Doppler indices of diastolic function demonstrate excellent intra- and interobserver reproducibility.[10] This is important when diastolic Doppler parameters must be compared with regional wall motion abnormalities in detecting myocardial ischemia.

1. *Early diastolic rapid filling* (E peak, cm/sec; E time-velocity integral, cm). During relaxation, there is a crossover (Fig. 6.8) between left atrial and left ventricular pressure, which causes the mitral valve to open and rapid filling to occur. The E wave results from the rapid filling phase (Figs. 7.16 and 7.17). In this part of

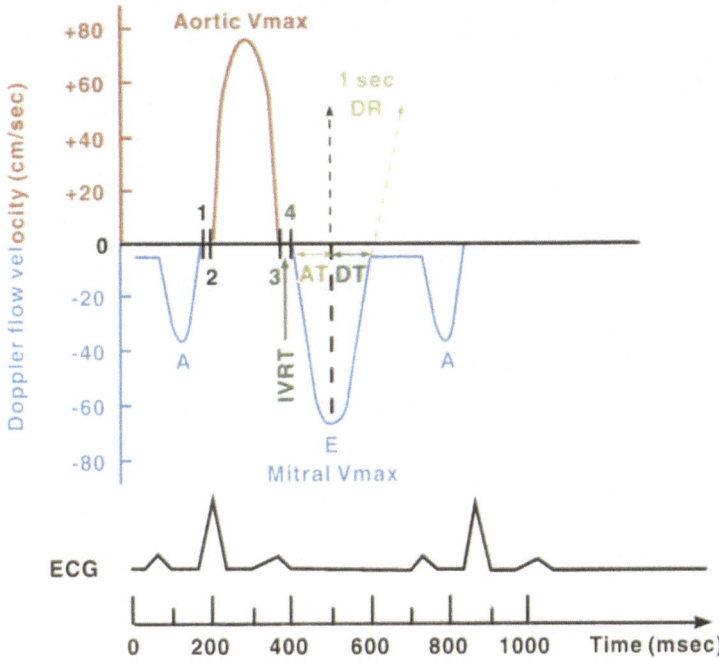

Fig. 7.16. Schematic representation of a recording of left ventricular outflow and mitral inflow with pulsed Doppler to measure the isovolumic relaxation time (*IVRT*). From a midesophageal view the sample volume is placed at an intermediate position between left ventricular outflow but in close proximity to the anterior mitral leaflet. *1* closure click of the mitral valve; *2* opening click of the aortic valve; *3* closure click of the aortic valve; *4* opening click of the mitral valve; IVRT laps between *3* and *4*; *E* early diastolic filling peak velocity; *A* atrial peak filling velocity; *AT* acceleration time; *DT* deceleration time; *DR* deceleration rate. *DR* is determined as the slope of a straight line drawn through the peak of the early diastolic filling flow signal to the end of the descending limb (in modern echocardiographic apparatus this information can be obtained in computerized form

the cardiac cycle left ventricular relaxation is still ongoing, causing a continuing drop in left ventricular pressure. The area under the E wave or thetime-velocity integral of the E wave (TVI), reflects the contribution of the rapid filling phase to left ventricular diastolic filling (rapid filling fraction). Moreover, early mitral diastolic filling rate appears to be an important parameter of ventricular performance (diastole is in dynamic relation to systole) since there is evidence that in patients with cardiogenic shock and unstable angina pectoris, intraaortic balloon pumping causes improvement in E despite a lack of improvement in ejection fraction.[11]

2. *Atrial peak filling velocity* (A peak, cm/sec, A time-velocity integral, cm), reflects the contribution of atrial contraction to the ventricular diastolic filling or atrial filling fraction (Figs. 7.16 and 7.17).

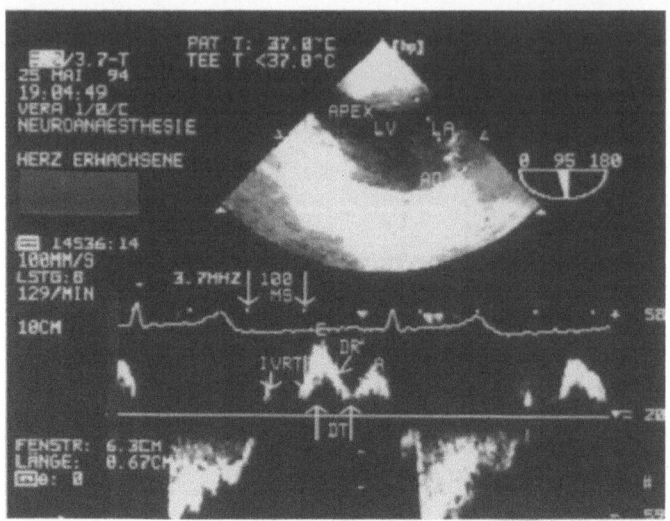

Fig. 7.17. Split-screen from two-dimensional midesophageal transverse plane (Top) and Doppler transmitral echocardiographic display from the same view (Bottom) demonstrating measurements of isovolumic relaxation time (IVRT). The Dopller sample volume is placed at an intermediate position between left ventricular outflow but in the proximity to the anterior mitral leaflet. The speed of the Doppler record is 100 mm/sec. *A* atrial diastolic peak filling; *AML* anterior mitral leaflet; *Ao* aortic outflow; *E* early diastolic peak filling; *LA* left atrium; *LV* left ventricle; *LVOT* left ventricular outflow tract

Table 7.7. Normal value of the Doppler transmitral flow parameters.

Measurements	Normal
E	78 ± 14 cm/sec
A	54 ± 12 cm/sec
E/A	1.45 ± 0.4
Deceleration time	198 ± 31 msec
Deceleration rate	4.2 ± 0.9 m/sec^2
IVRT	69 ± 12 msec

Data are from our laboratory.
E peak early diastolic filling wave; *A* peak atrial late diastolic filling wave; *IVRT* isovolumic relaxation time.

3. *E:A ratio* (units). This is the ratio between peak (or area) E and A and is commonly used to describe diastolic function.
4. *Isovolumic relaxation time* (IVRT in msec). This classical mechanocardiographic time interval[13,12] can be derived from Doppler tracing as a time lapse between

aortic valve closure click or the end of the Doppler aortic outflow signal to the mitral valve opening click or the onset of the E peak[1,3,7,9] (Figs. 7.16 and 7.17). IVRT reflects the speed of the initial part of left ventricular relaxation, which is a process requiring active energy and is further determined by end-systolic aortic pressure, the left atrial pressure at the time of mitral valve opening and by the elastic recoil of the myocardium. A prolonged IVRT is a sensitive marker of abnormal left ventricular relaxation in acute ischemia[3,12] as well as other chronic myocardial diseases (ventricular hypertrophy, hypertensive heart disease or hypertrophic cardiomyopathy).

5. *Deceleration rate* of the early diastolic peak filling (DR in m/sec^2). This parameter represents the speed of decrease of blood filling in the left ventricle after the peak E. It can be manually obtained by extrapolating the descending limb of the E wave starting from the peak until 1 sec of the tracing is reached (Fig. 7.16). Modern echocardiographs (Hewlett Packard) provide such calculations automatically.

6. Acceleration and deceleration time of the E wave and their measurements are given in Fig. 7.16. It should be pointed out that for heart rates beyond normal values of 60–80 beats per min all the above-mentioned time intervals must be corrected for heart rate according to Bazett's formula: corrected interval = measured interval$/\sqrt{R - R}$.

Practical remarks on measurement of Doppler transmitral parameters

The wall filter often obscures the initial point of upslope of the E wave on the time axis. This initial point may be identified either by extrapolating the relatively straight upslope of the E wave down to the baseline, or by dropping a vertical line from the origin of the velocity signal at the top of the wall filter. The former method has advantages, because it is independent of the wall filter setting and appears more representative of actual flow events. The point of mitral valve opening may occasionally be indicated by a click, which can be used to identify the time of onset of transmitral flow. Similar considerations apply to timing the cessation of the A wave.

The method used to separate the E and A waves in the absence of diastasis (by heart frequency more than 90–100 beats/min) have been similarly variable. The demarcation of the two waves in such situation can be done as follows. The end of the E wave may be considered as the point at which the two waves meet, and a vertical line dropped from that point to the baseline separates the waves adequately (Fig. 7.18). Others have considered that the A wave artificially truncated the E wave in this situation and have extrapolated the descending limb of the E wave down to the baseline to describe it, ignoring the A wave entirely. The A wave may then be considered as that portion of the velocity spectrum that remains, or it may be demarcated similarly by extrapolating its ascending limb to the baseline and ignoring the E wave entirely (Fig. 7.18).

Whichever method is used, the interpretation of measurements made when E and A waves merge is unclear and should be made very cautiously. It cannot be simply

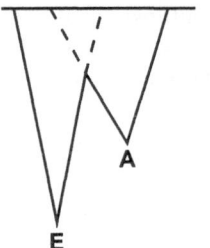 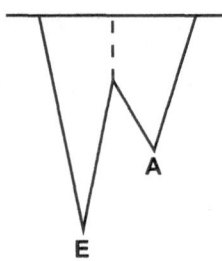

Fig. 7.18. Two various ways that may be used to demarcate the *E* and *A* waves

assumed that characteristics of the E and A waves can be measured meaningfully by extrapolating the inner side of the wave as though the other wave did not exist, because the two waves do not behave independently of one another.

Relation between mitral flow characteristic and hemodynamics

Transmitral Doppler velocity waveforms are determined by a complex interplay of a variety of hemodynamic and other factors. A discussion of all the factors that alter diastolic function is beyond the scope of this chapter. Nevertheless, it is important to recognize that diastole is a dynamic and complex phase of the cardiac cycle that depends on the proper interplay of multiple factors. These include (a) active myocardial relaxation; (b) the stiffness of the left ventricular chamber, which in itself depends on the passive elastic properties of the myocardium, the thickness of the ventricular wall, the interaction between the two ventricles; (c) transmitral pressure gradient; (d) loading conditions; (e) mitral valve function; and (f) intrathoracic pressure.

Special consideration has to be done for the effect of respiration and application of positive end-expiratory pressure. During inspiration the peak velocity of transmitral E wave, as well as A wave has been reported to decrease. The effects of respiration of flow velocities across the tricuspidal valve a quite opposite.[9] Because of the variation in transatro-ventricular flow velocities with respiration, the respiratory phase during Doppler recordings should be standardized and analysis should be made of beats taken during end-expiration.

Fig. 7.19 shows normal transmitral inflow (A) during ventricular diastole and the basic abnormal velocity patterns. The pattern "relaxation abnormality" (B) is seen in patients with impaired relaxation, such as in acute ischemia, i.e., E amplitude is decreased, atrial contribution to ventricular filling A is augmented, with E/A < 1, and IVRT is elongated, DT is increased and DR is decreased. In this situation, left ventricular end-diastolic pressure, left atrial pressure and pulmonary capillary wedge pressure (PCWP) are minimally increased.[3,7,13] The pattern "increased preload" (C) is characterized by a relative increase in E amplitude, E/A > 1 and normal IVRT.[7] This latter pattern can also be seen in patients with predominately increasing myocardial stiffness.[13,14] Actually, changes in preload have a major effect on compliance because of the curvilinear diastolic pressure-volume relationship. Increased preload will increase left atrial pressure relative to left ventricular pressure

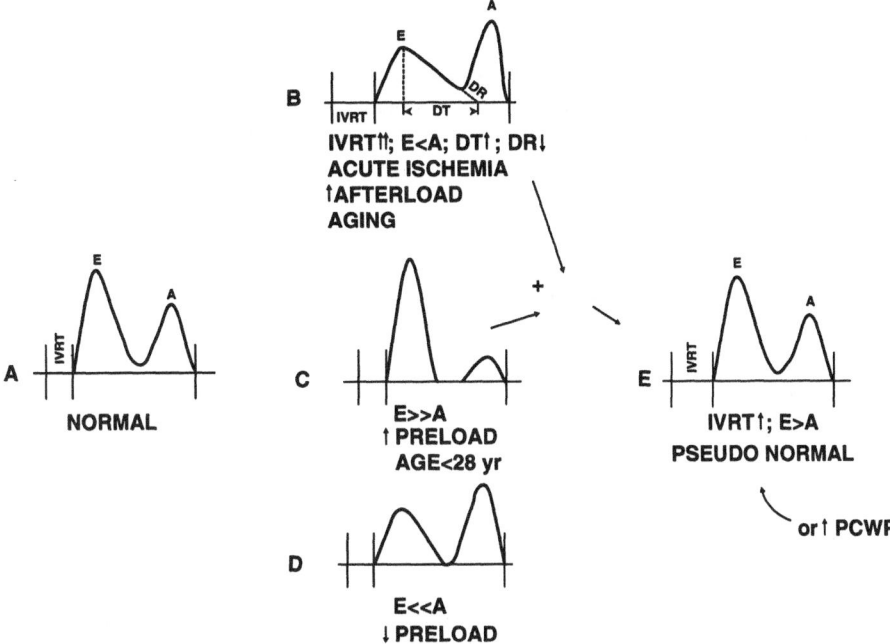

Fig. 7.19. Schematic representation of the patterns of Doppler transmitral inflow for evaluation of ventricular diastolic function and ischemia. See text for abbreviations and explanation

in early diastole, resulting in a higher driving pressure and thus a higher E wave with a rapid deceleration. Decreased preload (D) has the opposite effect. The mitral flow velocity profile has also been shown to change with age (aging slightly decreases peak E wave, increases peak A wave with augmentation of E/A ratio)[15] and heart rate (an increase of heart rate decreases peak A wave and hence reduces E/A ratio).[16,17]

Doppler transmitral flow for intraoperative diagnosis of acute myocardial ischemia

Experimental Doppler studies[18,19] in open-chest dogs have shown striking early abnormalities in left ventricular filling occurring after coronary artery occlusion. Fischer et al.[20] showed that changes in E/A ratio correlated well with negative dP/dt after proximal left anterior descending coronary artery occlusion. In humans, left ventricular diastolic dysfunction may be demonstrated by Doppler echocardiography both during acute ischemia as well as in patients with chronic CAD. Fuji et al.[21] demonstrated impaired filling patterns by Doppler echocardiography in acute myocardial infarction. Vissner et al.[22] have shown that E/A ratio correlates with cardiac risk index.

In an effort to evaluate acute transient myocardial ischemia, continuous recording of transmitral flow via transesophageal echocardiography during coronary angioplasty in humans has been performed,[23-25] demonstrating marked reversal of the E/A ratio within 15 seconds after balloon inflation. These Doppler-determined abnormalities of diastolic dysfunction *precede* the development of segmental wall motion abnormality, indicating that Doppler evaluation of transmitral flow may be an exquisitely sensitive and early marker of myocardial ischemia. Similar Doppler transmitral flow findings have been reported during bicycle exercise-induced angina pectoris,[8] spontaneous attacks of Prinzmetal's angina[26] or pacing-induced angina pectoris.[27] When there is reduced early filling, as there is in transient myocardial ischemia, the contribution of atrial contraction is generally enhanced, and this helps to maintain overall venous return and cardiac output.

The fact that myocardial relaxation consumes only 15–20% of high-energy phosphates raises the possibility that it is more sensitive to a low level of ischemia than systolic function and that mild myocardial ischemia may alter diastolic function without affecting systolic function.[28] The concept that diastolic dysfunction may precede systolic dysfunction suggests that impaired diastolic performance during ischemia may not only be the first manifestation of ischemia but may also contribute to further ischemia.[1] For example, impairment of isovolumic relaxation with reduction in the rate of decrease of early diastolic wall tension (as reflected by an augmented isovolumic relaxation period and decreased DR)[12] may impede regional antegrade coronary blood flow, since it is known that coronary supply takes place in early diastole (Fig. 7.20).

One practical question that every clinician should raise is, *Does Doppler transmitral flow provide additional independent confirmation about the presence of acute ischemia beyond that provided by SWMA?* In this context it must be mentioned that Doppler transmitral diastolic flow depends on the temporal pattern of pressure gradients across the mitral valve,[29] and thus it is determined not just by changes in relaxation and compliance. As the left atrial pressure rises, the velocity of flow across the mitral

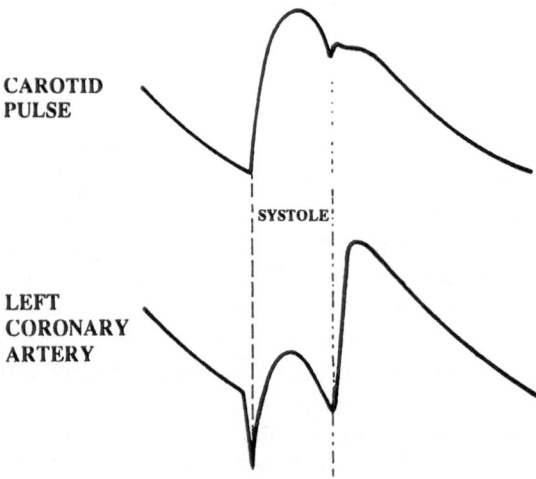

Fig. 7.20. Comparison of phasic blood flow in the left coronary artery and the systemic circulation (carotid pulse) during cardiac cycle

valve during atrial systole increases. As the left ventricular end-diastolic pressure itself increases, however, the difference in pressure across the valve becomes less pronounced.[17,30] This can result in apparent normalization of the mitral Doppler trace when both the ventricular and atrial pressures are elevated. This process is called "pseudonormalization" (Fig. 7.19E), and it represents the major obstacle to using the mitral E/A ratio as a parameter for myocardial ischemia.[31] Thus, before one can conclude that a patient is suffering acute ischemic events, two other causes of low E/A ratio must be excluded. The first is an acute pressure overload, in which the increase in left ventricular afterload results in a prolongation of the time constant of myocardial relaxation, such as with infusion of catecholamines. The second is a decrease in left ventricular preload.

The different mechanisms that can produce Doppler changes suggestive for ischemia limit the accuracy of a single measurement taken from the transmitral flow velocity. However, our result[32] suggest that the combining several measurements in a scoring system from 0 to 4 (Table 7.8) improves the diagnosis of myocardial ischemia.

To return to the question, "Does Doppler transmitral diastolic flow provide additional independent confirmation about the presence of acute myocardial ischemia beyond that provided by SWMA?" The answer is almost certainly *yes*, in some patients (patients with nonischemic causes for abnormal left ventricular segmental wall motion: bundle branch block, ventricular pacing, postischemic myocardial stunning, postcardiac surgery myocardial stunning, prosthetic valve, infiltrative disorder of the left ventricle) and under some conditions (no marked changes in pre- and afterload).[32]

Furthermore, perhaps of greater importance is that an appreciation of the concept of diastolic dysfunction in transient myocardial ischemia may alter the approach to this paramount problem, so that more complete efforts can be made to prevent recurrent ischemia, even if it is asymptomatic. In this context, medication with positive lusitropic effects such as calcium channel blockers[34] and particularly phosphodiesterase inhibitors,[34,35] may prove to be beneficial in the subset of patients with diastolic dysfunction. On contrary, failure to achieve a desired effect with specific therapy in an individual with acute transient ischemia may be secondary to an unfavorable change in left ventricular diastolic function.[1]

Table 7.8. Quantitative Doppler transmitral diastolic function scoring system (in the absence of mitral value lesions)

	DR (m/sec^2)	DT (msec)	IVRT (msec)	E/A (ratio)	Scores
Normal	3.3–5.1	170–230	57–81	1.05–1.85	0
Mild dysfunction	3.2–3.0	231–270	80–90	1.04–0.90	1
Moderate dysfunction	2.9–2.7	271–280	91–100	0.91–0.81	2
Severe dysfunction	2.6–2.4	281–290	101–110	0.80–071	3
Extreme dysfunction	< 2.4	> 290	> 110	< 0.7	4

Source: Our laboratory.

References

1. Kolev N, Zimpfer M. Impact of myocardial ischemia on diastolic function. Clinical relevance and recent Doppler echocardiographic insights. Eur J Anaesth 11(in press), 1994
2. Braunwald E, Sonnenblick EH, Ross J Jr. Mechanisms of cardiac contraction and relaxation. In: Braunwald E ed, Heart disease, 4th ed. WB Saunders, Philadelphia, pp 370–373, 1992
3. Roelandt JRTC,. Principles of Doppler assessment of diastolic left ventricular function. In: Roelandt JRTC, Sutherland GR, Iliceto S, Linker DT, eds. Cardiac ultrasound. Churchhill Livingstone, Edinburgh, London, pp 233–239, 1993
4. Apstein CS, Grossman W. Opposite initial effects of supply and demand ischemia on left ventricular diastolic compliance: the ischemia diastolic paradox. J Mol Cell Cardiol 19: 119–128, 1987
5. Iskandrian AS, Heo J, Segal BL, Askenase A. Left ventricular diastolic function: Evaluation by radionuclide angiography. Am Heart J 115: 924–929, 1988
6. Pearson AC, Nelson J, Kanter J. Effect of sample volume location on pulsed Doppler-evaluation of leftventricular filling. Am J Cardiac Imaging 2: 40–45, 1988
7. Quinones MA. Doppler assessment of left ventricular diastolic function. In: Nanda NC, ed. Doppler echocardiography, 2nd ed. Lea & Febiger, Philadelphia, pp 197–215, 1993
8. Kolev N. Assessment of left ventricular function in ischemic heart disease using pulsed Doppler transmitral flow during exercise. J Cardiovasc Diag Proc (NY) 11: 15–18, 1990
9. Huemer G, Kolev N, Kurz A, Zimpfer M. Influence of positive end-expiratory pressure on right and left ventricular performance assessed by Doppler two-dimensional echo-cardiography. Chest 106: 67–73, 1994
10. Galderisi M, Benjiamin EJ, Eraus JC. Intra- and interobserver reproducibility of Doppler assessed indexes of left ventricular diastolic function in a population-based study (the Framingham Heart Study). Am J Cardiol 70: 1341–1345, 1992
11. Iskandrian AS, Hakki AH, Heo J, Bemis CE, Kane S, Mandler J. Effect of intraaortic balloon pumping on left ventricular ejection fraction, systolic ejection rate and peak filling rate. J Appl Cardiol 1: 271–283, 1986
12. Kolev N, Romoda T. Clinical value of calibrated and differentiated displacement apexcardiography in ischemic heart disease. Cardiology (Basel) 69: 343–352, 1982
13. Appleton CP, Hatle LK, Popp RL. Relation of transmitral flow velocity patterns to left ventricular diastolic function: new insights from a combined hemodynamic and Doppler echocardiographic study. J Am Coll Cardiol 12: 426–430, 1988
14. Nishimura RA, Abel MD, Hatle LK, Tajik AJ. Relation of pulmonary vein to mitral flow velocities by transesophageal Doppler echocardiography. Effects of different loading conditions. Circulation 81: 1488–1497, 1990
15. Zoghbi WA, Habib GB, Quinones MA. Doppler assessment of right ventricular filling in a normal population: Comparison with left ventricular filling dynamics. Circulation 82: 1316–1320, 1990
16. Downes TR, Nomeir A, Stewart K. Effect of alteration in loading conditions on both normal and abnormal patterns of left ventricular filling in healthy individuals. Am J Cardiol 65: 377–381, 1990
17. Mulvagh S, Qinones MA, Kleiman NS, Cherif J, Zoghbi WA. Estimation of left ventricular end-diastolic pressure from Doppler transmitral flow velocity in cardiac patients independent of systolic performance. J Am Coll Cardiol 20: 112–119, 1992
18. Pandin N, Funai J, Wang SS, Lowell B. Effect of regional ischemia on diastolic left ventricular flow vortex – color Doppler and contrast echocardiographic studies. J Am Coll Cardiol 7: 147A–151A, 1986
19. Rinder ML, Courtis MR, Perez JE, Brasiliai B, Ludbrook PA. Alterations in Doppler indexes of diastolic function following coronary artery reperfusion. Circulation 74II: 47–53, 1986

20. Fischer DC, Voyles W, Sikes W, Greene ER. Left ventricular filling patterns during ischemia: An echo/Doppler study in open chest dogs. J Am Coll Cardiol 5: 426A–431A, 1985

21. Fujii J, Yazaki H, Sawada H, Aizawa T, Watanabe H, Kato K. Noninvasive assessment of left ventricular diastolic filling in ischemic heart disease. J Am Coll Cardiol 5: 1155–1160, 1985

22. Vissner CA, Koning H, Delmarre B, Koolen JJ, Dunning AJ. Pulsed Doppler derived mitral inflow velocity in acute myocardial infarction: An early prognostic indication. J Am Coll Cardiol 7: 136A–141A, 1986

23. Labovitz AJ, Lewen MK, Kern M, Vandormael M, Deligional U, Kennedy HL, Habermechl K, Morsek D. Evaluation of left ventricular systolic and diastolic function during transient myocardial ischemia produced by angioplasty. J Am Coll Cardiol 10: 478–755, 1987

24. De Bruyne B, Lerch R, Meyer B, Schlaepfer H, Gabathauer J, Rutischause W. Doppler assessment of left ventricular filling during brief coronary occlusion. Am Heart J 117: 629–634, 1989

25. Wind BE, Sinder AJ, O'Neill WW, Topol EJ, Dilworth RL. Pulsed Doppler assessment of left ventricular filling in coronary artery disease before and immediately after coronary angioplasty. Am J Cardiol 59: 1041–1046, 1987

26. Moscarelli E, Distante A, Rovai D, Lombardi M, Morals A. Changes in mitral flow induced by transient myocardial ischemia in man. Circulation 74II: 230–237, 1986

27. Iliseto S, Amico A, Marangelli V. Doppler echocardiographic evaluation of pacing-induced ischemia on left ventricular filling in patients with coronary artery disease. J Am Coll Cardiol 11: 953–961, 1989

28. Iskandrian AS, Jaekyeong H, Segal BL, Askenase A. Left ventricular diastolic function: Evaluation by radionuclide angiography. Am Heart J 115: 924–928, 1986

29. Appleton CP, Gonzales MS, Basnight MA. Relationship of left atrial pressure and pulmonary venous flow velocities: Importance of baseline mitral and pulmonary venous flow velocities patterns studied in lightly sedated dogs. J Am Soc Echocardiogr 7: 264–275, 1994

30. Appleton CP, Hatle LK. The natural history of left ventricular filling abnormalities: assessment by two-dimensional and Doppler echocardiography. Echocardiography 9: 437–457, 1992

31. Nishimura RA, Abel MA, Tajik AJ. Assessment of diastolic function of the heart: background and current applications of Doppler echocardiography. Part II. Clinical studies. Mayo Clin Proc 64: 181–204, 1989

32. Huemer G, Kolev N, Spiss CK, Zimpfer M. Comparison of Doppler transmitral diastolic parameters and systolic wall motion abnormalities during perioperative myocardial ischemia (Abstr). Anesthesiology 81: A105, 1994

33. Elkayam U, Amin J, Mechra A, Vaques J, Weber L, Rachimtoola SH. A prospective, randomized double-blind, crossover study to compare the efficacy and safety of nifidipine therapy with that of isosorbide dinitrate and their combination in the treatment of ischemic heart disease and congestive heart failure. Circulation 82: 1954–1961, 1990

34. Krams R, McFalls E, Van der Giessen WJ, Serruyis PW, Verdoun PD, Roelandt J. Does intravenous milrinone have a direct effect on diastolic function? Am Heart J 121: 1951–1955, 1991

35. Klocke RK, Mager G, Kux A, Hopp HW, Hilger HH. Effects of a twenty-four-hour milrinone infusion in patients with severe heart failure and cardiogenic shock as a function of the hemodynamic initial condition. Am Heart J 121: 1965–1973, 1991

Myocardial perfusion by contrast echocardiography: new trend in ischemia detection (scenario of the year 2000)

Until recently, in cases of myocardial ischemia cardiac ultrasound offered no methods of evaluating myocardial perfusion other than assessment of the end results of ischemia, that is, detection of wall motion abnormalities. This technique requires dysfunctional myocardial tissue to detect underlying tissue ischemia and does not provide a true measurement of the extent of nonviable myocardial tissue. Over the past decade, myocardial contrast echocardiography has been developed as a technique with the potential to fill this void. By injecting sonographic contrast agent into animals whose circumflex coronary artery had been occluded, it was possible to single out ischemic areas more accurately than waiting for the onset of segmental wall motion abnormalities.[1] Further, this way of identifying areas at risk has proven to be highly specific, reproducible, and does not require complicated reference systems as in systolic wall motion analysis.

Principles of contrast echocardiography

Myocardial contrast echocardiography is an evolving technique that can be used to assess myocardial perfusion in vivo. It uses the intravascular injection of micro-bubbles of air, which produce contrast enhancement when passing through the myocardium during simultaneously performed two-dimensional echocardiography. The source of myocardial ultrasound contrast effect, as it relates to clinically produced contrast, is *microbubbles* contained in the injected solution.[2,3] These form discrete ultrasound targets within the blood pool that have the same velocity and distribution as their neighboring red blood cells. Microbubbles, because they represent an interface between liquid or tissue and gas, are an exceptionally strong ultrasound reflector. Thus, myocardial contrast effect is presumed to be due to the presence of microbubbles flowing to the arteriolar or capillary bed and hence increasing the ultrasound reflectance of the myocardium. Reflective intensity of the microbubbles is proportional to their concentration in the blood pool of myocardium. The absolute size of the microbubbles (6–30 microns, which is approximately 1/2 of the ultrasound wavelength used), within limits, is probably less of a factor in determining the contrast effect intensity than is the absolute number of bubbles.[4]

Presently, there are mainly two types of ultrasonic contrast agents, namely, free and encapsulated gas bubble. The earliest ultrasound contrast agents were produced by *manual agitation* of a liquid such as normal saline, dextrose, sodium diatrizoate (Renografin), etc. This shaking generated air bubbles that would serve as echo reflectors. However, it was observed that manually prepared bubbles were variable in size and in persistence. Therefore, the potential for air emboli existed. Further, due to their relatively large size and transience (prone to rapid coalescence), the microbubbles were not very useful for visualizing myocardial structures after intravenous injections. The method was improved by the subsequent use of a sonicator to create smaller and stable microbubbles. *Sonication* as a method for generation of echocontrast agents consists of applying high-frequency (20 KHz) ultrasonic energy on a carrier solution, with simultaneous introduction of a small amount of air into the solution.

The technology now most often used requires either intracoronary or aortic root injection for myocardial visualization.[3,5] As such, its uses are limited to the catheterization laboratory and the operating room at the time of coronary artery bypass surgery or balloon dilatation. By peripheral venous injection, microbubbles are either trapped by the pulmonary vasculature or decay before their appearance in the left heart.[6] Nevertheless, the development of agents capable of transpulmonary transit in high concentrations after venous application is underway.[7–12] Albunex® (Molecular Biosystems Inc, San Diego, CA), a commercially prepared solution of sonicated albumin, has a mean diameter of 4 μm with 95% of the particles under 10 μm and is supplied in 4 ml vials in concentrations of 300 to 500 million particles/ml. A second contrast agent, Echovist,® SHU 508 (Schering AG Lab., Berlin, Germany) is a hyperosmolar preparation of nonencapsulated microbubbles (99% < 8 μm) that is prepared by suspending a solid saccharide (galactose) precursor in water. Because of the relatively large dimensions of the microbubbles of sonicated Renographin-76, dextrose, and sorbitol solutions as compared with capillary size and their associated hyperosmolarity, these agents are not optimal absolute quantitative contrast agents. The associated hyperosmolarity of the latter agents may lead to a hyperemic response and thus alter native flow patterns or cause alterations in the contractile state of the myocardium.

Another significant issue in attempting to identify myocardial perfusion is that of microvascular physiology. The covarying aspects of tissue blood flow and blood volume can be detected using contrast echocardiography today. However, tissue blood flow and tissue blood volume are not directly or linearly related. Recent studies have shown that coronary anatomy (as defined by angiography) may not adequately indicate myocardial perfusion or tissue viability and thus, visual interpretation of coronary angiograms does not predict the physiologic importance of coronary stenosis.[6] Today, a primary clinical issue is the relation between coronary anatomy and myocardial perfusion. To illustrate this point, Fig. 7.21 highlights the discrepancy between epicardial coronary vessel diameter and coronary flow. The studies of Ito et al.[14] showed that myocardial perfusion and epicardial coronary anatomy are not interchangeable as markers of predicting tissue viability. This is shown symbolically in Fig. 7.21, where the branches of the tree represent coronary anatomy and the leaves of the tree represent tissue perfusion. As can be seen in this diagram, the tree may have normal branches but no leaves (indicating no perfusion), even when the underperfused branch otherwise appears to be normal. Although considerably more complex, the coronary anatomy of the patient may appear to be normal and yet may have abnormal or inadequate myocardial perfusion. The converse may also be true; that is, one may have abnormal coronary anatomy (coronary stenoses or occlusions) and yet maintain adequate perfusion. Because the human coronary anatomy, as assessed by

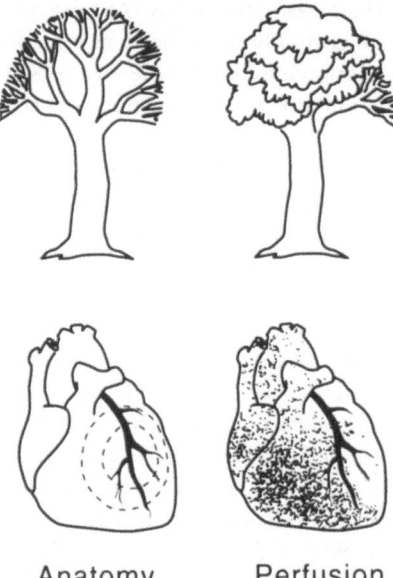

Anatomy   Perfusion

Fig. 7.21. This symbolic diagram represents the apparent differences between anatomy and perfusion. In the tree model, it is observed that the anatomy (branch) may be intact, yet the perfusion is lacking. By comparison, in the heart model, it is possible to have abnormal coronary anatomy and yet the degree of the myocardial perfusion may remain unknown

angiography, has not been shown to predict the myocardial perfusion pattern uniformly, the use of contrast echocardiography as a perfusion marker may now play a significant role in the management of patients having acute or chronic exacerbated myocardial ischemia.[15]

Quantitative analysis of myocardial contrast two-dimensional echocardiography

Along with the development of new echocardiographic contrast agents, the quantitative analysis of myocardial contrast images also requires that new two-dimensional echocardiographic technique be developed. This is because the echocardiographic contrast effect is related to an increase in the video intensity of the images. Computerized video densitometric analysis of the myocardial echo intensities during contrast appearance and disappearance must also be developed. It might be useful to recall that a two-dimensional echocardiographic scan plane has an actual thickness, called the elevation (Fig. 7.22). A videodensity measurement in a region of myocardium therefore reflects, because of this elevation, a videodensity value in a corresponding volume of myocardium, including blood-containing tracer.[5] After the injection of a sonographic contrast agent, the myocardial videodensity will therefore reflect the amount of contrast present in a certain volume of myocardium. Basically, two different types of measurements can be obtained, namely, changes in flow due to changes in tissue blood volume and/or changes in tissue transit time.

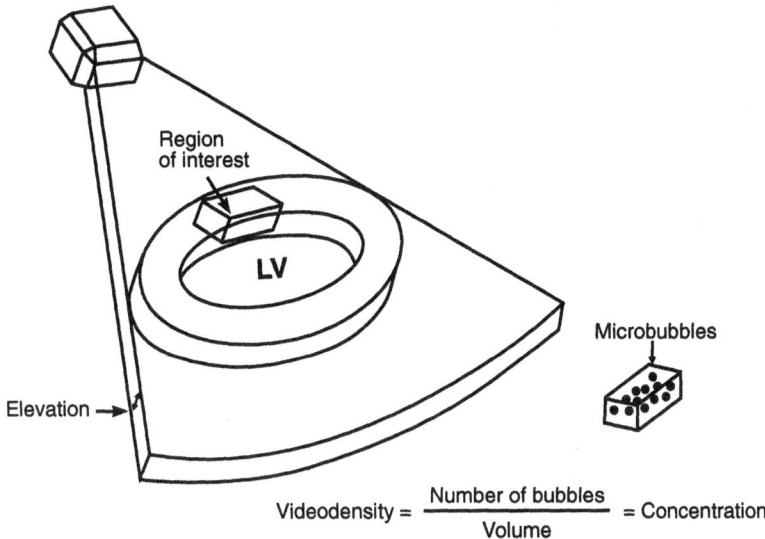

$$\text{Videodensity} = \frac{\text{Number of bubbles}}{\text{Volume}} = \text{Concentration}$$

Fig. 7.22. Stylized representation of left ventricular (*LV*) cross-sectional thickness by TEE. Tissue characterization via myocardial contrast echocardiography provides measurements of the myocardial concentration of a contrast agent (microbubbles). Since a two-dimensional scan plane has an actual thickness, called the elevation, the myocardial videodensity reflects the amount of contrast medium (microbubbles) in a certain volume of myocardium, including blood containing tracer

(a) Assessment of the perfusion territory or regional myocardial perfusion mapping

Microbubbles in a coronary artery serve as a marker of blood flow distribution within the perfusion territory of the artery. By comparing the echo intensity of the image in different myocardial areas at one and the same time of the cardiac cycle (diastole, because coronary flow take place in diastole and during systole there is marked reduction in myocardial contrast due to collapse of the microbubbles[16]) one obtains *measurement of the "risk area,"* i.e., myocardial perfusion. Determination of the perfusion territory of an occluded vessel is based solely on whether or not the myocardium distal to a coronary stenosis or occlusion demonstrated opacification following injection of contrast. In the case of myocardium jeopardized by acute ischemia, the region supplied from the affected coronary artery will have a lower concentration of microbubbles and hence lower brightness or "acoustic contrast drop out" (Fig. 7.23). Risk area determined by contrast echocardiography has been shown to compare favorably with that measured by both intracoronary injection of colored dyes and technetium autoradiography.[17] The high resolution of myocardial contrast echocardiographic images facilitated separation of normal and ischemic zones, permitted the recording of risk area in multiple tomographic planes from which the three dimensional extent of the perfusion bed could be serially determined.

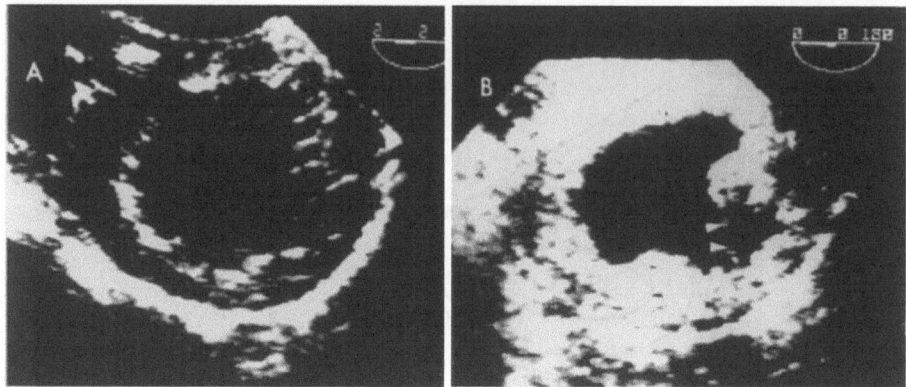

Fig. 7.23. Two-dimensional left ventricular short-axis view at the level of the papillary muscles (A) before injection of a contrast medium. (B) the postcontrast image shows an ischemic myocardium that is not contrast enhanced, i.e., "acoustic contrast drop out" (demonstrated by arrowheads)

Actually, risk area can be defined using contrast echocardiography as (a) the area failing to show contrast enhancement when contrast is injected proximal to the site of occlusion ("negative" risk area) or (b) the area demonstrating contrast enhancement when the contrast agent is injected directly into the coronary artery immediately distal to the site of occlusion ("positive" risk area). The spatial extent of risk area measured using these two approaches differs slightly[18]. When other variables such as perfusion pressure in the nonoccluded bed are within the physiologic range, the "positive" risk area is larger than the "negative" area[19]. In the experimental canine model, the difference between the two areas is predominantly in their epicardial extent[19].

The same relationship has been observed using other techniques for assessment of risk area and has been studied in detail by injecting colored dyes into coronary vessels at and proximal to the site of occlusion.[20] The risk area defined by direct injection of dye just distal to the site of occlusion reflects only antegrade perfusion and does not include collateral flow. This risk area has been defined as the anatomic risk area,[20] and the positive risk area on myocardial contrast echocardiography, therefore, is the in vivo equivalent of the anatomic risk area. When dye is injected proximal to the site of occlusion, the unstained region is the area not supplied by either antegrade flow or collateral flow through adjacent vessel. The risk area defined in this manner has been termed the functional risk area[20]. The negative risk area defined by contrast echocardiography, therefore, is the in vivo equivalent of the functional risk area. Depending of the extent of collateral flow, the functional riskarea will invariably be smaller than the anatomic risk area.[21]

In a canine model of total coronary occlusion where collateral flow to the occluded bed was increased in increasing collateral driving pressure, diminution in the size of the contrast echocardiographically defined perfusion bed was noted.[22] In patient with chronic CAD there are abundant collaterals, and these vessels are present in both the epicardium and endocardium. This has not generally been appreciated, because there are no appropriate methods of assessing collateral blood flow in humans. Most collateral vessels are < 100 μm in diameter, and coronary angiography, the most commonly employed technique for assessing the coronary circulation, can only detect vessels > 100 μm in diameter.[23] Several factors contribute to the improved visualization of collateral flow using contrast echocardiography. First, because contrast echocardiography uses microbubbles whose size is similar to that of red blood sells, it should be possible to identify collateral flow in humans that might otherwise be inapparent. Second, after right coronary artery bypass, a pressure gradient develops between the right coronary artery and the left anterior descending arterial bed, which could open collapsed collateral vessels. Third, cardioplegia results in vasodilation, which may further enhance collateral blood flow. Myocardial contrast echocardiography, therefore, has the potential for assessing the interaction between risk area, collateral flow, and myocardial viability.

Recent studies demonstrated a close relation of risk area to the extent of SWMA[18] Assuming that the extent of regional dysfunction correlates with the size of the risk area, one could argue that the region of dysfunction alone could be used to determine the size of the ischemic zone. There are several reasons for independently determining risk area. First, although the region of dysfunction correlates with infarct size, the precision of separation between ischemic and nonischemic zones does not approach the resolution that can be attained using contrast. Second, although a discrete coronary occlusion can be performed in the canine model, in clinical situation SWMA can be present in beds other than those supplied by the acutely occluded artery. These beds could represent either old infarction, postischemic ("stanned") myocardium, or chronically ischemic ("hibernating") myocardium.[24] Because no established patterns of SWMA can reliably differentiate between these possible causes of abnormal motion, the size of the risk area cannot be definitely established using SWMA alone. Finally, in addition to being influenced by the analytical technique applied, the relationship between the region of dysfunction and the ischemic/infarcted zone varies with time after occlusion and is independently affected by preload and afterload,[25] while myocardial contrast echocardiography appears to be more suitable measure of the area at risk.

What are the relationship between risk area and hemodynamics? Experimental data suggest that when cardiac output and left ventricular ejection fraction are normalized to baseline values, each is inversely and linearly related to risk area. However, without normalization, this relationship is not apparent.[25] Cardiac output and left ventricular ejection fraction cannot, therefore, be used reliably in the clinical setting to determine the size of the risk area during acute myocardial ischemia. For example, a left ventricular ejection fraction of 0.50 may represent a drop of 0.15 in a patient with a baseline ejection fraction of 0.65 but may represent a normal left ventricular ejection fraction in another patient. In addition, when risk area is < 18% of the left ventricular myocardium, the left ventricular ejection fraction may not change, which is due to compensatory hyperkinesis of other normally perfused regions.[26] In contrast to cardiac output and ejection fraction, mean arterial pressure may even rise above baseline during acute myocardial infarction, which may reflect arterial vasoconstriction that is due to catecholamine response. It is only when risk area is very large ($> 40\%$ of the left ventricular myocardium) that arterial pressure starts to decline.

Using contrast echocardiography estimation of risk area offers another avenue for the intraoperative assessment of the adequacy of myocardial perfusion. During CABG surgery, flow of cardioplegia solution through the coronary circulation may be impaired by coronary stenosis.[27] Insufficient cardioplegia delivery to the regions of the myocardium supplied by stenotic coronary arteries could cause inadequate myocardial protection, resulting in ischemia or infarction. Depending on the sensitivity of the technique used to detect myocardial infarction, perioperative infarction can occur in 5 to 20% of all bypass operations.[28] If region of the myocardium most susceptible to ischemic injury could be identified, the vessels supplying these regions could be bypassed first and cardioplegia delivered earlier; potentially lessening the chance of perioperative infarction.

At present, perioperative coronary angiography provides the cardiac surgeon and anesthetist with a road map to estimate the degree and location of coronary arterial stenosis. They are thus able to judge where to place bypass grafts to achieve successful revascularization. Coronary angiography, however, frequently does not accurately assess the anatomic[29] or the physiologic[30] significance of coronary artery stenosis, which has led to the development of other intraoperative techniques for assessing anatomy and blood flow. For example, high resolution intraoperative epicardial echocardiography is capable of imaging coronary arteries and bypass graft anastomosis to evaluate the degree of coronary arterial stenosis and the technical success of a bypass graft.[31] Intraoperative Doppler flow probes can also be used to measure bypass graft blood flow to region of myocardium.[32] With neither of these techniques, however, it is possible to evaluate multiple perfusion beds simultaneously. Both methods require manipulation of the heart during operations. Furthermore, they do not provide information regarding either collateral flow or total nutrient flow.

Contrast echocardiography has several potential advantages over these techniques: It allows the physician to measure the size of myocardial perfusion beds, it can be used to determine perfusion to different regions of the myocardium simultaneously; and, it can delineate the degree of collateral flow to underperfused myocardial zones. During CABG operations, cardioplegia is delivered to the cross-clamped aortic root through a cannula at controlled flow rates to reduce myocardial temperature and to produce cardiac arrest in order to achieve myocardial preservation. The ideal time to perform contrast echocardiography is during cardioplegia delivery, because delivery of contrast through the aortic root is possible without interfering with the surgical routine and repetition of contrast echocardiography is possible during each dose of cardioplegia, allowing data acquisition at baseline and after completion of each distal coronary anastomosis. Practically, microbubbles of known sizes have been introduced into the cardioplegia solution and have become the principal means of assessing myocardial perfusion during operation.[33]

Retrograde cardioplegia is now used intraoperatively during bypass surgery allowing to perfuse regions of the myocardium supplied by severely stenosed vessels, which may not receive adequate cardioplegia after aortic root injection. No intraopertive method, however, assesses the intramyocardial distribution of retrogradely delivered cardioplegic solution. This is important because the balloon on the coronary sinus catheter, which is inflated during cardioplegia delivery, has a tendency to obstruct venous tributaries draining into the sinus. A method for assessing the intramyocardial distribution of cardioplegia solution could permit the position of the balloon to be readjusted. Unlike the situation when contrast is injected into the aortic root, contrast is readily noted, even when epicardial coronary arteries are occluded.[34] Myocardial contrast echocardiography could, therefore, provide clues to the ideal method of cardioplegia (antegrade vs retrograde) in patients with severe multivessel disease, in whom intraoperative myocardial perfusion may be an issue.

For myocardial contrast echocardiography to be used as a routine clinical tool in noncardiac surgery patients or in ICU it is imperative that myocardial contrast enhancement be achieved following a *peripheral* venous injection of contrast. Recent studies indicate that this may become a reality in the near future. Right atrial injection of sonicated albumin has been demonstrated to reproducibly opacify the left ventricular myocardium in dogs.[35-37] It is possible to highlight subtle changes in signal intensity produced by myocardial contrast echocardiography by displaying intensity levels in color rather than black and white because the human eye can appreciate only 16 gray levels but can discriminate several hundred color hues.[16]

(b) Qualification of regional myocardial blood flow

The ultrasonic backscatter from any myocardial region is increased proportionally to the amount of echocontrast agent present within this region. As the echocontrast bolus arrives in a myocardial region, the ultrasonic backscatter increases, while during the washout period it decreases again to the baseline level. These changes of backscatter during the contrast transit time are measured as digitized video-intensity. Thus, the sampling of data in contrast echocardiography requires a precise temporal synchronization and quantitation of regional myocardial blood flow is far more difficult than simply defining the perfusion territory of a coronary vessel.

The steps involved in quantitation of myocardial perfusion during contrast echocardiography are data acquisition, selection of appropriate frames, alignment of these frames and placement of the region of interest to derive time-inensity plot. A digital echocardiographic system with a broad range (120 db) and at least 250 levels of gray would be desirable for data acquisition. Because such a system is not commercially available, analog data from the video output port of the echo system can be sent directly to a computer for on-line analysis. Because coronary blood flow occurs in diastole, and because end-diastolic frames are easy to identify, they have been conventionally used to generate time-intensity plots. This can be done by employing a gating device (i.e., an R-wave trigger) to select end-diastlolic frames. For the purpose a region of interest is defined in a reference frame that is approximately equal to the area within the epicardial outline.

Briefly, by plotting the time intensity of brightness versus time, one obtains time-intensity curves. The algorithm for analyzing the time-intensity curves are, in general, adapted from indicator dilution theory. Contrast echocardiographic time-intensity curve have a relatively steep upward slope, followed by a peak and then a slower, less steep, downward part (Fig. 7.24). By assuming that the downward sloping part of the curve is monoexponential, it is possible to calculate the intensity half-life $(t_{1/2})$ by means of the formula:

$$t_{1/2} = \ln 2/k$$

where k is the coefficient of the curve obtained by logarithmically interpolating the downward slope. This type of calculation can give *an assessment of coronary stenosis and myocardial blood flow*. $t_{1/2}$ was calculated for normal flow conditions and in the case of an induced stenosis of 85% and a coronary occlusion; in each condition, in order, $t_{1/2}$ was significantly greater.[38] Data have been generated in vivo by comparing myocardial time-intensity curve parameters to myocardial blood flow measured using radiolabelled microshperes.[39] In one such study, microbubbles and radiolabelled microspheres were injected into the left circumflex coronary artery at varying flow rates using a different label for each flow. In this experiment contrast appears in the fourth end-diastolic frame, reaches maximal intensity by the eighth frame, and gradually disappears.

Over the last few years there have been numerous scientific presentations on contrast echocardiographic time-intensity curves. However, the data found in the literature are rather discordant. When the variation in the time-intensity curve peak have been compared with the variations in coronary flow, either positive correlations[40] or no correlations[13] have been found. Thus, analysis of the time-intensity curve has not yet given satisfying results for the quantitation of myocardial perfusion by contrast ehcocardiography.

The limitations regarding quantitation of myocardial perfusion by means of contrast echocardiography may not necessarily compromise a sufficient evaluation of the coronary reserve in clinical practice. To this end it is enough for an echocardiographic parameter to present variations of the same size as the variations of the coronary flow in order to be able to discriminate those cases in which the incapacity of the coronary to vary within a wide range is indicative of a reduced

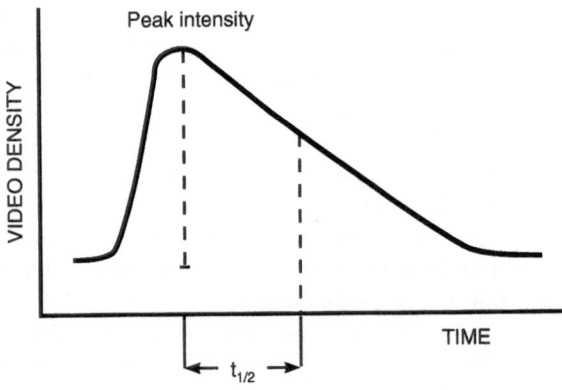

Fig. 7.24. Time-intensity curve obtained during a contrast myocardial perfusion study

coronary reserve. Cheirif et al.[40] have evaluate the variations of the peak contrast intensity after intracoronary injection of papaverine in 40 patients and found that an increase in peak intensity not above 10 units was 80% sensitive and 29% specific for coronary artery disease. Other investigators[41] have carried out a quantitative analysis of the time-intensity curves, before and after papaverine intracoronary injection, obtained from the echocardiograms performed in dogs in which a critical stenosis had been created on a coronary branch. The area under the curve, peak intensity and curve width did not correlate with absolute blood flows measured with radiolabelled microsphere. However, the ratios of the areas under the curves, derived from the "normal" and "hypoperfused" vascular bed, respectively, correlated well with the ratios of blood flows in the same myocardial region during each stage of the experiment. Thus, myocardial contrast echocardiography seems to be able to differentiate the regions with normal increase in myocardial flow (obtainable with powerful coronary vasodilators) from those supplied from a critically stenosed coronary in which there is no such increase. The accuracy of this evaluation still has to be tested: most experiments have been conducted on animals in whom it is possible to ascertain the increase of myocardial flow objectively. The lack of a true gold standard of measurement of the coronary reserve in humans makes it difficult to check the validity of the method in the clinical context. The presence of numerous variables which can affect the time-intensity curve call for caution in analysing the experimental results; for example, the time-intensity curve is affected by the blood's velocity as well as by the intravascular volume; vasodilator agents can affect these two parameters differently and often not in a way that can be predicted.[42]

Conclusion

The qualification of myocardial perfusion by means of contrast echocardiography is exciting and challenging. Several promising early studies have provided insightful information as to the future of this modality for studying myocardial tissue viability, assessing risk area and regional blood flow. The demonstration that myocardial opacification can be achieved following right atrial injection of contrast in experimental animals raises hopes that this technique can be used clinically following peripheral venous injection of contrast. If this proves to be the case, the technique should find a much broader clinical application in the noninvasive assessment of regional myocardial perfusion in patients suspected or known to have coronary artery disease. In this regard, enhancements in bubble engineering, optimization of echocardiographic imaging systems (greater sensitivity and dynamic range) and the availability of digital image-enhancement techniques will be required for myocardial contrast echocardiography to realize its full clinical potential by the year 2000.

References

1. Shapiro JR, Xie F, Meltzer RS. Myocardial contrast two-dimensional echocardiography: Dose-myocardial effect relations of intracoronary microbubbles. J Am Coll Cardiol 12: 765–771, 1988

2. Keller MK, Segal SS, Kaul S, Duling B. The behavior of sonicated albumin micro-bubbles within the microcirculation: a basis for their use during myocardial contrast echocardiography. Circ Res 65: 458–463, 1989

3. Meltzer RS, Amico AF, Reisner SA, Shapiro JR. Contrast agents for myocardial perfusion studies: Mechanisms, state of the art and future prospects. In: Iliceto S, Rizzon P, Roelandt JRTC, eds. Ultrasound in coronary artery disease. Kluwer, Dordrecht, pp 351–363, 1991

4. Halmann M, Beyar R, Rinkevich D, Shapiro JR, Sidemann S, Markiewicz W, Meltzer RS, Reisner SA. Digital subtraction myocardial contrast echocardiography: Design and application of a new analysis program for myocardial contrast perfusion imaging. J Am Soc Echocardiogr 7: 355–362, 1994

5. Rovai D, L'Abbate A. Application of indicator dilution principles to perfusion imaging. In: Roelandt JRTC, Sutherland GR, Iliceto S, Linker DT, eds. Cardiac ultrasound. Churchill Livingstone, Edinburgh, pp 513–551, 1973

6. Feinstein SB. Myocardial perfusion: Contrast echocardiography perspectives. Am J Cardiol 69: 36H–41H, 1992

7. Wiencek JG, Feinstein SB, Walker R, Aronson S. Pitfalls in quantitative contrast echocardiography: the steps to quantitation of perfusion. J Am Soc Echocardiogr 6: 395–416, 1993

8. Heidenreich PA, Wiencek JG, Zaroff JG. In vitro calculation of flow using contrast ultrasonography. J Am Soc Echocardiogr 6: 51–61, 1993

9. Rovai D, Ghelardini G, Trivella MG. Difference between myocardial transit time of sonicated albumin microspheres and radionuclide labelled albumin (Abstr). Eur Heart J 12 [Suppl]: 221, 1992

10. Walker R, Wiencek JG, Aronson S. The influence of intravenous Albunex injection on pulmonary hemodynamics, gas exchange, and left ventricular peak intensity. J Am Soc Echocardiogr 5: 462–470, 1992

11. Rasmussen CM, Mizoguchi AH, Markovitz PA, Bruns DE, Armstrong WF, Dittrich HC. Albunex during dobutamine stress echocardiography: improved transpulmonary passage and lowered dose requirements (Abstr). J Am Soc Echocardiogr 7: 1A, 1994

12. Mor-Avi V, Cholley B, Robinson K, Ng A, Sandelsky J, Marcus R, Lang RM, Shroff S. Albunex microspheres and left ventricular contractility: load and heart rate independent analysis using an isolated rabbit heart (Abstr). J Am Soc Echocardiogr 7: 31B, 1994

13. Kaul S. Clinical application of myocardial contrast echocardiography. Am J Cardiol 69: 36H–41H, 1992

14. Ito H, Tomooka T, Sakai N, Yu H, Higashino Y, Fujii K, Masuyama T, Kitabatake A, Minamino T. Lack of myocardial perfusion immediately after successful thrombolysis. A predictor of poor recovery of left ventricular function in anterior myocardial infarction. Circulation 85: 1699–1705, 1992

15. Lim YJ, Nanto S, Masuyama T, Kodama K, Ikeda T, Kitabatake A, Kamada T. Visualization of subendocardial myocardial ischemia with contrast echocardiography in humans. Circulation 79: 233–244, 1989

16. Melzer RS, Ohad D, Reisner S, Sucher E, Kaplinsky E, Motro M, Battler A, Vered Z. Quantitative myocardial ultrasonic integrated backscatter measurements during contrast injections. J Am Soc Echocardiogr 7: 1–8, 1994

17. Sakamaki T, Tei C, Meerbaum S, Shimoura K, Kondo S, Fishbein MC, Y-Rit J, Shah PM, Corday E. Verification of myocardial contrast two-dimensional echocardiographic assessment of perfusion defects in ischemic myocardium. J Am Coll Cardiol 3: 34–38, 1984

18. Kemper A, O'Boyle JE, Sharma S, Cohen CA, Cloner RA, Kituri S, Parisis AF. Hydrogen peroxide contrast-enhanced two-dimensional echocardiography: real time in-vivo determination of regional myocardial perfusion . Circulation 68: 603–6011, 1983

19. Kaul S, Pandian NC, Weymann AE. Contrast echocardiography in acute myocardial ischemia: I. In-vivo determination of total left ventricular "area at risk." J Am Coll Cardiol 6: 825–830, 1985

20. Marcus ML. Effects of corornary occlusion on myocardial perfusion. In: The coronary circulation in health and disease. McGraw-Hill, New York, p 221, 1993

21. Jugdutt BI, Hutchins GM, Bulkley BH, Becker LC. Myocardial infarction in the conscious dogs: three dimensional mapping of infarct, collateral flow, and region at risk. Circulation 60: 1141–1147, 1979

22. Kaul S, Pandian NG, Weyman AE. The effects of selectively altering the collateral driving pressure on regional perfusion and function in the occluded coronary bed in the dogs. Circ Res 61: 77–83, 1987

23. Cohen MV. Morphological consideration of the coronary collateral circulation in man. In: Coronary collaterals. Clinical and experimental observations. Futura, New York, pp 1–11, 1985

24. Smucker ML, Beller GA, Watson DD, Kaul S. Left ventricular dysfunction in excess of the size of infarction: a possible management strategy. Am Heart J 115: 749–754, 1988

25. Wyatt WH. Contrasting effects of alterations in ventricular preload and afterload upon systemic hemodynamics, function, and metabolism of ischemic myocardium. Circulation 55: 318–324, 1975

26. Kaul S, Glasheen W, Ruddy TD, Pandian NG, Weyman AE, Okada RD. The importance of defining left ventricular area at risk in vivo during acute myocardial infarction: an experimental evaluation with myocardial contrast two-dimensional echocardiography. Circulation 75: 1249–1260, 1987

27. Grondin CM, Helias J, Vouhe PR, Robert P. Influence of a critical coronary artery bypass stenosis on myocardial protection though cold potassium cardioplegia. J Thorac Cardiovasc Surg 82: 608–613, 1981

28. Massie BM, Mangano DT. Assessment of perioperative risk: have we put the card before the horse? J Amer Coll Cardiol 21: 1353–1356, 1993

29. Braunwald E, Sobel BE. Coronary flow and myocardial ischemia. In: Braunwald E, ed. Heart disease, 4th ed. WB Saunders, Philadelphia, pp 1161–1197, 1992

30. Khuri SF. Intraopertaive assessment of the physiological significance of coronary stenosis in humans. J Thorac Cardiovasc Surg 92: 71–78, 1986

31. Hiratzka LF. Inrtraoperative evaluation of coronary artery bypass graft anastomoses with high frequency epicardial echocardiography: experimental evaluation and initial patient studies. Circulation 73: 1199–1204, 1986

32. Greene ER, Reilly PR, Myrands IP, Doppler ecocardiographic assessment of the left internal mamary grafts in humans (Abstr). Circulation 74 [Suppl 2] II: 308, 1986

33. Aronson S, Lee BK, Wiencek JG, Feinstein SB, Roizen MF, Karp RB, Ellis JE. Assessment of myocardial perfusion during CABG surgery with two-dimensional transesophageal contrast echocardiography. Anesthesiology 75: 433–440, 1991

34. Villanueva PS. Assessment of myocardial distribution of coronary sinus retrograde cardioplegia using myocardial contrast echocardiography. Circulation 82 [Suppl 3] II: 26, 1990

35. Villanueva. Successful and reproducible myocardial opacification during two-dimensional echocardigraphy from right heart injection of contrast. Circulation 85: 1557–1562, 1992

36. Amico AF, Iliceto S, Saponetti LS, Memmola C, Rizzon P. Myocardial contrast echocardiography for the evaluation of coronary flow reserve. In: Illiceto S, Rizzon P, Roelandt JRTC, eds, Ultrasound in Coronary Artery Disease. Kluver, Dordrecht, pp 389–393, 1991

36a. Meza MF, Greener Y, Perry B, Hunt R, Bales G, Revall S, Murgo JP, Cheirif J. Myocardial contrast echocardiography: successful transpulmonary myocardial opacification in a canine model of occlusion-perfusion (Abstr). J Am Soc Echocardiogr 7 [Suppl 2]: S2, 1994

37. Dittrich HC. Bales GL; Hunt RM, McFerran BA, Kuvelas T, Widder KJ, Greenr Y. Myocardial perfusion by intravenously administrated novel ultrasound contrast agents in canine (Abstr). J Am Soc Echocardiog 7 [Suppl 2]: S36, 1994
38. Kaul S, Kelly P, Oliver JD, Glasherrn WP, Keller MW, Watson DD. Assessment of regional myocardial blood flow with myocardial contrast two-dimensional echocardiography. J Am Coll Cardiol 8: 143–149, 1986
39. Takeuchi M, Araki M, Nakashima Y, Kurowa A. Comparison of dobutamine stress echocardiography and stress thallium-201 single-photon emission computed tomography for detecting coronary artery disease. J Am Soc Echocardiogr 6: 593–602, 1994
40. Cheirif J, Zoghbi WA, Raizner AE, Minor ST, Winters WL, Klein MS, DeBauche TL. Lewis JM, Roberts R, Quinones MA. Assessment of myocardial perfusion in humans by contrast echocardiography. I. Evaluation of regional coronary reserve by peak contrast intensity. J Am Coll Cardiol 11: 735–743, 1988
41. Keller MW, Glasheen W, Smucker ML, Burwell LR, Watson DD, Kaul S. Myocardial contrast echocardiography in humans. II. Assessment of coronary blood flow reserve. J Am Coll Cardiol 12: 925–934, 1988
42. Reisner SA, Shapiro JR, Amico AF, Meltzer RS. Myocardial contrast echo washout curves: the influence of ischemia and hyperemia (Abstr). J Am Coll Cardiol 13: 115, 1989

Subject index*

---

* Pages numbers followed by f indicate figures: those followed by t indicate tables.

Alexander Aloy, Eva Schragl

Jet-Ventilation

Technische Grundlagen und klinische Anwendungen

1995. 126 Abbildungen. VIII, 184 Seiten.
Broschiert DM 76,–, öS 532,–
ISBN 3-211-82551-7

Das vorliegende Buch stellt erstmals das gesamte Spektrum der normo- und hochfrequenten Jet-Ventilation dar. Nach der Darstellung der experimentellen Grundlagen und Überlegungen zum Wirkungsmechanismus werden die einzelnen Formen der Jet-Ventilation, die Applikationsmöglichkeiten und die gebräuchlichen Jet-Respiratoren im Detail beschrieben. Der zweite Teil des Buches behandelt die klinischen Einsatzmöglichkeiten der Jet-Beatmung, sowohl intraoperativ (mikrolaryngeale- und Thoraxchirurgie, Bronchoskopie und Stentimplantation) als auch in der Intensiv- und Notfallmedizin. Ein eigenes Kapitel ist dem Einsatz in der Pädiatrie gewidmet. Es wird weiters auf das Monitoring eingegangen, hämodynamische Auswirkungen, mögliche Komplikationen und die Grenzen der Jet-Ventilation werden kritisch beleuchtet.
Das Buch soll Anästhesisten, Intensivmedizinern und Pulmologen als Nachschlagwerk und praktischer Ratgeber für den Einsatz dieser speziellen Beatmungsform dienen.

Preisänderungen vorbehalten

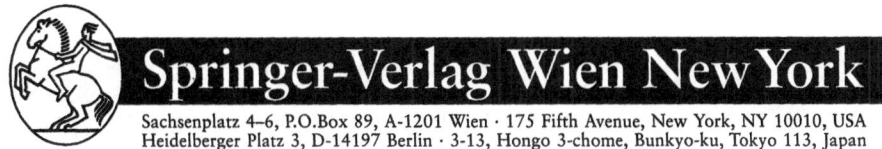

Springer-Verlag Wien New York

Sachsenplatz 4–6, P.O.Box 89, A-1201 Wien · 175 Fifth Avenue, New York, NY 10010, USA
Heidelberger Platz 3, D-14197 Berlin · 3-13, Hongo 3-chome, Bunkyo-ku, Tokyo 113, Japan

G. Kleinberger, K. Lenz, R. Ritz, H.-P. Schuster,
G. Simbruner, J. Slany (Hrsg.)

Beatmung

1993. 16 Abbildungen. VII, 145 Seiten.
Broschiert DM 49,–, öS 345,–
ISBN 3-211-82438-3
(Intensivmedizinisches Seminar, Band 5)

Die respiratorische Insuffizienz stellt eines der zentralen Probleme des Patienten auf
der Intensivstation dar. Durch Verbesserung der Technik in der maschinellen
Beatmung und in den augmentierenden Verfahren sowie in der medikamentösen
Therapie ist es in den letzten Jahren gelungen, große Fortschritte in der Behandlung
dieser Patienten zu erzielen. In diesem Band sind die wichtigsten Vorträge der 11.
Wiener Intensivmedizinischen Tage, deren Hauptthema die Beatmung war,
dargestellt. Neben der Pathophysiologie der Beatmung wird die Therapie bei den
verschiedenen Ursachen der respiratorischen Insuffizienz abgehandelt. Es werden
hierbei die verschiedenen Formen der Beatmung und die medikamentösen Therapien,
wie die Applikation des Surfactant beim Frühgeborenen und beim Erwachsenen
sowie die NO Therapie beim Patienten mit ARDS dargestellt. Weiters werden das
Für und Wider der Hämofiltration als unterstützende Therapie und die extra-
korporale CO_2 Elimination diskutiert. Insgesamt soll dieses Buch den aktuellen Stand
der wichtigsten Therapiemöglichkeiten bei der respiratorischen Insuffizienz sowie
praktisch relevante Information für den Intensivmediziner bieten.

Preisänderungen vorbehalten

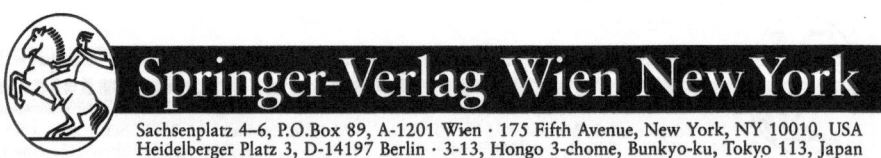
Springer-Verlag Wien New York
Sachsenplatz 4–6, P.O.Box 89, A-1201 Wien · 175 Fifth Avenue, New York, NY 10010, USA
Heidelberger Platz 3, D-14197 Berlin · 3-13, Hongo 3-chome, Bunkyo-ku, Tokyo 113, Japan

Springer-Verlag
and the Environment

WE AT SPRINGER-VERLAG FIRMLY BELIEVE THAT AN international science publisher has a special obligation to the environment, and our corporate policies consistently reflect this conviction.

WE ALSO EXPECT OUR BUSINESS PARTNERS – PRINTERS, paper mills, packaging manufacturers, etc. – to commit themselves to using environmentally friendly materials and production processes.

THE PAPER IN THIS BOOK IS MADE FROM NO-CHLORINE pulp and is acid free, in conformance with international standards for paper permanency.